HOW TO BE SUGAR FREE AND KEEP YOUR FRIENDS

HOW TO BE SUGAR FREE AND KEEP YOUR FRIENDS

Recipes by Megan Davies

PHOTOGRAPHY BY KIM LIGHTBODY

Hardie Grant

QUADRILLE

Introduction

Trying to remove such a widely and heavily used group of ingredients from your diet... and 'having a life' can be a real challenge, there's no doubt. There is, however, a generally very simple fix when it comes to cooking at home without refined sugars, with some simple habits to develop when it comes to shopping.

There is a plethora of delicious and flavoursome food out there that doesn't have (or simply doesn't need) the inclusion of refined sugars. The recipes in this book will help you ditch them, using instead some of the many natural sugars and sweeteners available that act as brilliant swap-ins and substitutes, leaving you just as satisfied, less 'bouncing off the wall then crashing' and certainly better health-wise too.

Too much refined sugar can increase your chance of developing heart disease, Type 2 diabetes, and encourages weight gain and acne... to name a few. We all know it's bad for our teeth, and that too much refined sugar (and therefore a bad diet, with lots of processed food) can cause havoc with energy levels and mental health.

One thing to note, though, is that sugar is sugar (whether it is refined or unrefined); it'll all get absorbed straight into the bloodstream once consumed, raise your blood sugar (though at varying speeds and durations depending on its glycemic index), and while it's great to treat yourself and enjoy sweet foods, balance, like everything in life, is key to a healthy lifestyle.

This book focuses on meals that would usually include refined sugar, but the amount of sugar or sweetness has been reduced as much as possible and, most relevantly, the types of sugar have been converted to non-refined sugars, all of which are natural.

A big part of reducing refined sugars in your diet is just focusing on eating unprocessed, unrefined foods as a whole. Easier said than done, but hey, you've got to start somewhere.

Xylitol, though it sounds pretty chemical, is a natural sweetener made from a variety of tree barks (and some veg too). It's the ingredient that looks, tastes and works most like caster (superfine) or granulated white sugar. This has been used in some of the dessert recipes to achieve as much of a similar outcome as one would have when using refined sugar. I've also used lots of coconut sugar. It looks and tastes more like a muscovado sugar, but make sure you pass it through a sieve as some hardy boulders can appear, which you want to avoid when adding to a cake mix, for example. Elsewhere, you'll see natural syrups like maple, agave or date syrup, all of which are brilliant unrefined ingredients. Honey is a great option, and is also used.

A lot of the sweetness throughout the recipes has been extracted from cooking with fruit and sweet vegetables, taking advantage of their natural flavour and fructose, while also giving you vitamins and nutrients! Make sure the fruit you use is at its ripest, so that you benefit from the ingredient at its sweetest stage (and therefore from its moisture too, particularly in baking).

In terms of cacao and chocolate (and with all-natural sweeteners), make sure you read the ingredients on the packet to ensure they are all natural: raw cacao with no refined sugar added! There are some great products out there. You'll be able to find some brand advice throughout the recipes.

Bircher Muesli

\\

SERVES 4

20g / 1 tbsp runny honey
2 apples, roughly chopped
2 tbsp water
200g / 2 cups porridge oats
100ml / 7 tbsp apple juice
60g / 2oz dried fruit, anything
   larger than raisins chopped
200ml / ¾ cup full-fat milk,
   plus extra to serve (cow's or
   plant-based, your choice)
1 cinnamon stick
1 pear
fresh fruit, seeds and Fruit
   Compote (page 27)
   (optional), to serve

Add the honey and apples to a small saucepan with the water. Bring to the boil, then reduce the heat to a gentle simmer for about 10 minutes, so the apples turn into a half-stewed state: softened but their structure still intact. Remove from the heat and set aside to cool to lukewarm.

Add the oats, apple juice, dried fruit, milk and cinnamon stick to a bowl and mix to combine. Add the lukewarm apple, mixing well to cool down further.

Cover, transfer to the fridge and leave to soak for at least 1 hour, or overnight.

Once you're ready to eat, remove the cinnamon stick and grate in the pear. Mix well and serve with a generous extra splash of milk, fresh fruit, seeds and Fruit Compote, if you like.

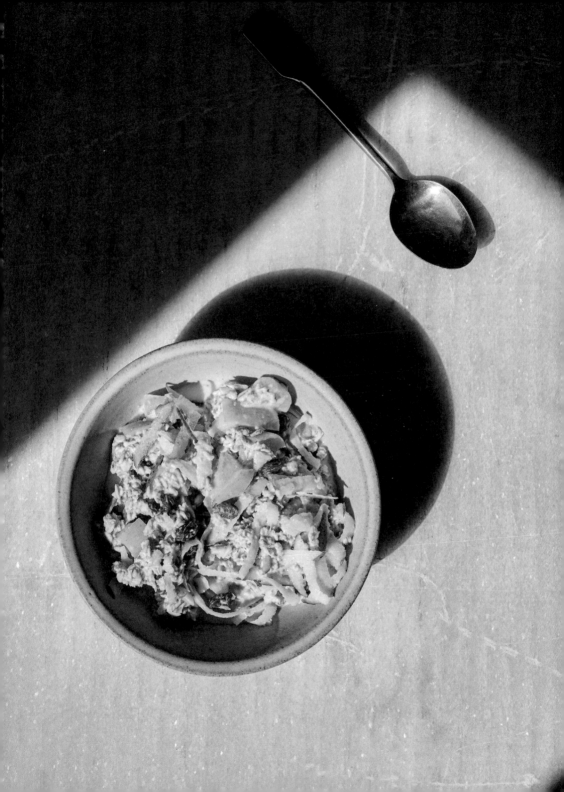

Spiced Granola

\\

MAKES 10–12 PORTIONS

250g / 2½ cups porridge oats

1 tbsp rapeseed (canola) oil

1 tbsp sesame oil

4 tbsp honey

½ tsp vanilla extract

80g / 3oz mixed seeds

80g / 3oz mixed nuts, roughly
  chopped

½ tsp ground cinnamon

½ tsp ground allspice

¼ tsp nutmeg, grated

80g / 3oz dried fruit (your
  choice, or a mix)

60g / 1¼ cups coconut flakes

Preheat the oven to 160°C / 320°F / gas mark 3.

Add all the ingredients apart from the dried fruit and coconut flakes to a large mixing bowl and mix very well to combine. Spread onto a large baking tray (pan) – or 2 if it's too crowded.

Bake for 40 minutes, tossing the mixture every 10 or so minutes. Add the dried fruit and coconut flakes, toss to combine and bake for another 10 minutes.

Once the granola is done, let it cool completely on the tray(s) without touching it, as you'll loosen any clumps; mix up once cool.

Store in an airtight container for up for 2 weeks.

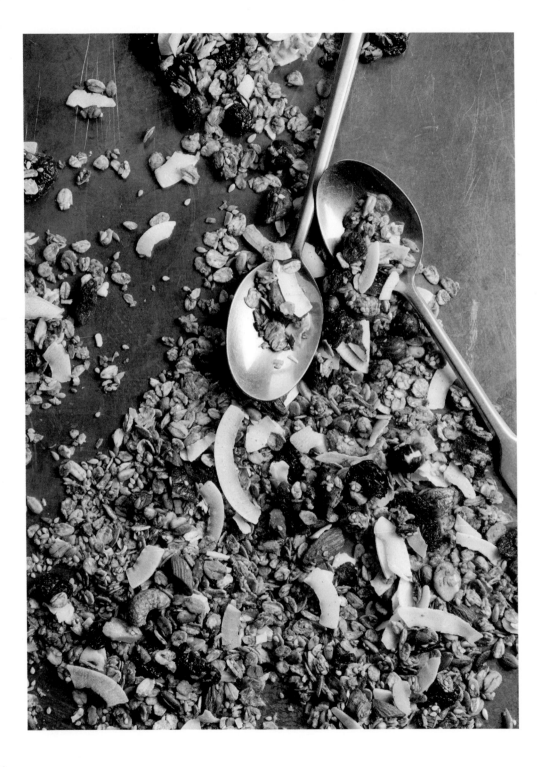

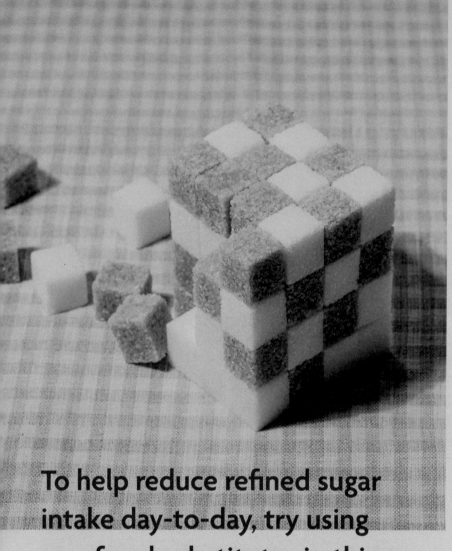

To help reduce refined sugar intake day-to-day, try using unrefined substitutes in things like tea, coffee, porridge or other savoury recipes where you might add a spoonful of sugar.

It's amazing how you can gradually cut out most (if not all) refined sugar from your diet without really realizing, once you have the unrefined alternatives at your fingertips.

Orange, Pear & Pecan Porridge

SERVES 4

2 oranges

2 pears

1 tbsp olive oil

pinch of sea salt, plus extra
  to serve

30g / ⅓ cup pecans

200g / 2 cups porridge oats

1.4l / 6 cups full-fat milk
  (or water if you like)

date syrup (optional),
  to serve

Preheat the oven to 220°C / 425°F / gas mark 7.

Using a sharp knife, segment the oranges over a bowl
to catch the juice and place the segments in the bowl.
Squeeze the remaining pith of the segmented oranges
over the segments in order to extract every bit of juice.

Slice the pears into discs and add to a small baking tray
(pan). Drizzle with half the saved orange juice from the
bowl, the oil and salt, then bake on the top shelf of the
oven for 10 minutes. Add the pecans to the tray and bake
for another 10 minutes.

Meanwhile, add the oats and milk to a saucepan and
gently bring to a boil, then let simmer for 10–15 minutes,
stirring constantly until cooked.

Transfer to bowls and top with the baked pears and
pecans, orange segments and the remaining orange juice.
Finish with an extra pinch of sea salt and a drizzle of date
syrup, if you need some more natural sweetness.

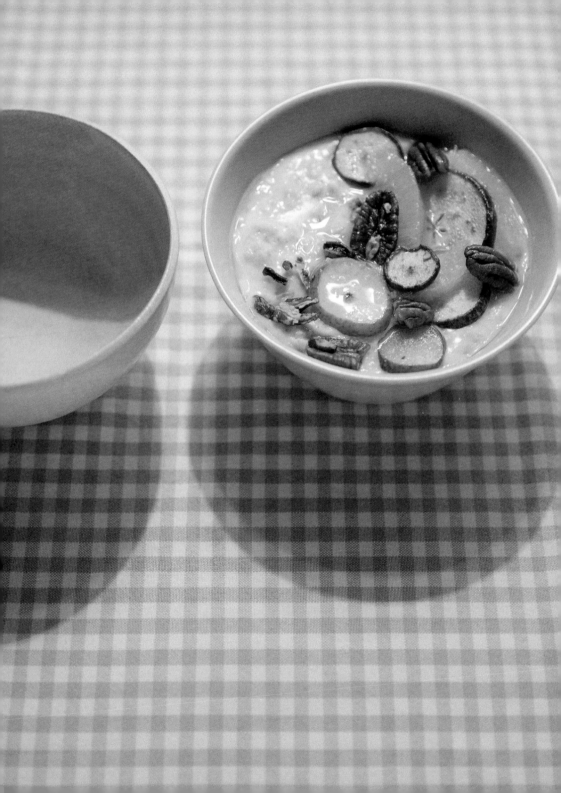

Peanut Butter & 'Jam' on Toast

SERVES 4

250g / 9oz frozen mixed
  berries (best to avoid too
  many blackberries or it'll
  be super-tart)

3 tbsp water

1 tsp pomegranate molasses

1 tsp date syrup

¼ tsp sea salt

4 slices of bread

4 tbsp crunchy peanut butter

Add the frozen berries and water to a small saucepan on a low heat and let defrost and break down for 5 minutes, stirring often. Once they are soft and bubbling, stir in the pomegranate molasses, date syrup and salt, and increase the heat slightly to a stronger bubble for 1 minute, stirring constantly. Remove from the heat.

Toast the bread slices.

Spread the peanut butter onto the toast, followed by the 'jam'. Best served with a strong coffee.

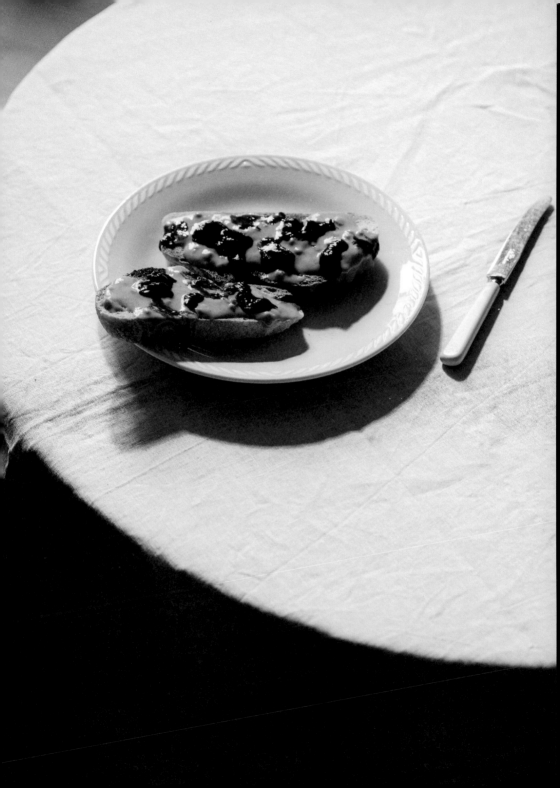

Coconut French Toast

SERVES 2

2 eggs

½ x 400g / 14oz can coconut milk

2 tbsp coconut sugar, sifted

pinch of sea salt

4 slices of bread (your choice)

40g / 1 cup coconut flakes

coconut oil, for frying

coconut yoghurt and ground cinnamon, to serve

Preheat the oven to 120°C / 250°F / gas mark ½.

Add the eggs, coconut milk, coconut sugar and salt to a large bowl. Whisk with a fork to combine, then add a slice of bread to the mixture to soak, turning it occasionally.

Place a large, non-stick frying pan over a low–medium heat, add the coconut flakes and toast for a couple of minutes (keep an eye on them so they don't burn), then transfer them to a small bowl.

Add a knob of coconut oil to the pan and let it melt.

Transfer the soaked slice of bread to the pan, and place a second slice in the bowl to soak as you fry the French toast for 3–4 minutes, or until golden brown. Carefully turn the slice over and fry for 3–4 minutes on the other side. Transfer to the oven, covered, to keep warm, and repeat with the remaining slices of bread.

Slice the cooked French toast slices in half and divide between plates, piling dollops of yoghurt on top and finishing with the toasted coconut flakes and a pinch of ground cinnamon.

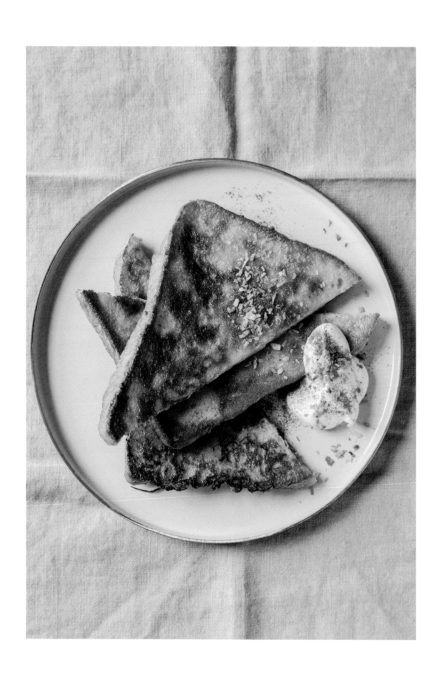

Fig & Tahini Muffins

\\\\\\\\\\\\\\\\\\\\\\\\\\\\\\\\\\\

MAKES 12 MUFFINS

250g / 1¾ cups plus 2 tbsp
  self-raising (self-rising)
  flour
60g / generous ½ cup ground
  almonds
1 tsp baking powder
80g / scant ½ cup coconut
  sugar, sifted
80g / ⅓ cup plain yoghurt
80g / 4 tbsp tahini (sesame
  paste)
3 eggs
2 bananas, mashed
4 fresh figs, trimmed and
  roughly chopped
1 tbsp sesame seeds

Preheat the oven to 200°C / 400°F / gas mark 6.

Place 12 muffin cases in the cavities of a 12-hole muffin tray (pan) and set aside.

Add the flour, ground almonds, baking powder and coconut sugar to a large mixing bowl, and the yoghurt, tahini (sesame paste), eggs and bananas to another bowl. Mix both (separately) to combine well, then add the wet ingredients to the dry, along with the figs, folding everything together to combine, while avoiding overworking the mixture.

Divide the mixture evenly between the muffin cases and sprinkle over the sesame seeds.

Bake on the top shelf of the oven for 25–30 minutes until risen and cooked through, then transfer the muffin tray to a cooling rack and leave for 5 minutes. Remove the muffins in their cases from the tray and leave to cool completely.

Serve or store in an airtight container for up to 3 days, or in the freezer for up to 1 month.

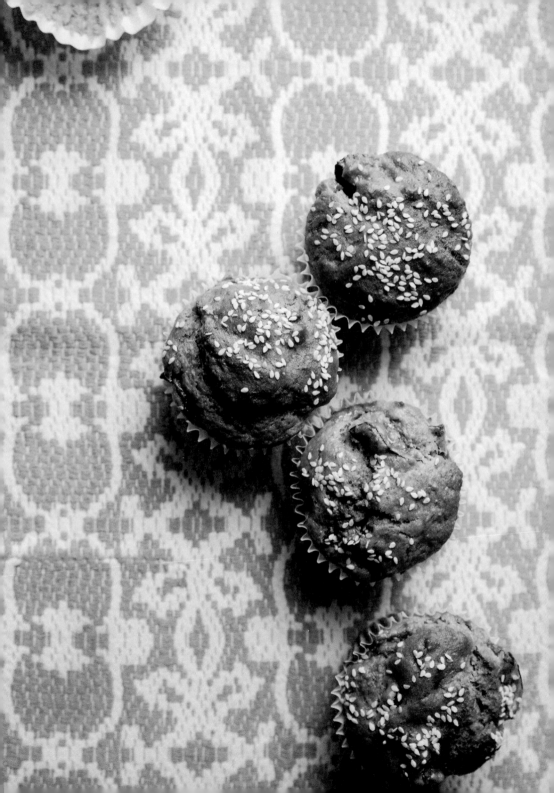

Breakfast Shortcake Cookies

MAKES 6 COOKIES

100g / ¾ cup self-raising
  (self-rising) flour, plus extra
  for dusting
50g / ½ cup porridge oats
½ tsp baking powder
50g / 1¾oz xylitol
¼ tsp sea salt
80g / ⅓ cup butter, chilled
  and diced
1 egg
40ml / 3 tbsp buttermilk
  (or plain yoghurt and a
  squeeze of lemon juice)
½ banana, thinly sliced
salted butter or yoghurt,
  to serve

Preheat the oven to 190°C / 375°F / gas mark 5. Line a large baking tray (pan) with parchment paper.

Add the flour, oats, baking powder, xylitol and salt to a food processor and blitz briefly until combined, then add the butter and process until the mixture resembles breadcrumbs. Next, add the egg and buttermilk and briefly pulse until you have a sticky dough.

Tip out onto a clean, lightly floured work surface and bring the dough together with your hands. Pull a handful of dough off and roll into a rough ball, avoiding working it too much. It's a very wet mix, but just go with it. Place on the lined baking tray and repeat with the remaining mixture, spacing the balls well apart, to make 6 in total.

Place a couple of slices of banana in the centre of each ball, overlapping them slightly, and press down gently to slightly flatten the ball. Bake on the top shelf of the oven for 20 minutes until slightly risen and cooked through (a skewer should come out clean). Let cool for 5 minutes on the tray, then transfer to a cooling rack.

Serve with salted butter, the remaining banana and some yoghurt, or just as they are with a coffee.

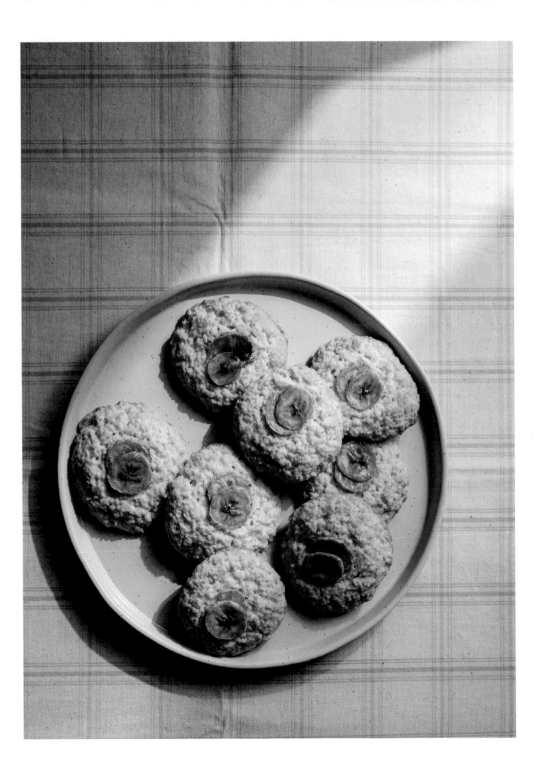

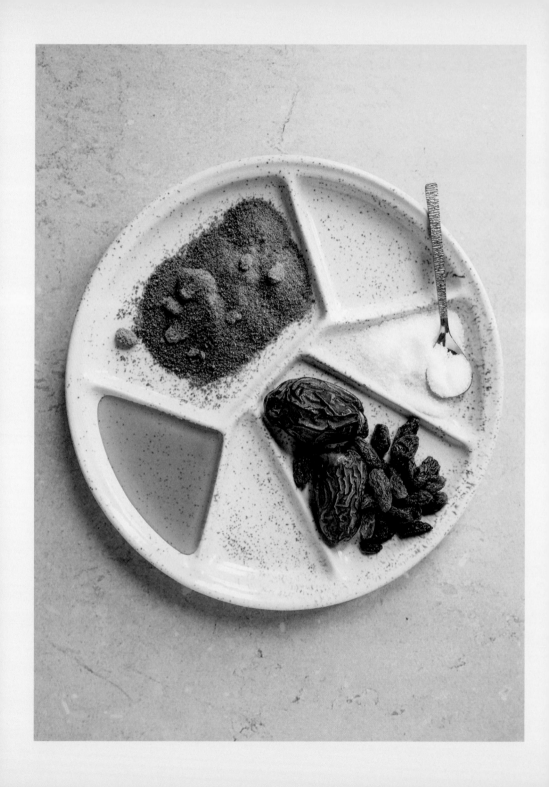

Refined sugar substitutes are now easy to get hold of in large supermarkets. Be sure to add these to your shopping list for cooking ease:

/ agave nectar
/ coconut sugar
/ honey
/ maple syrup
/ date syrup
/ xylitol

Homemade Nutella

MAKES 200ML / ¾ CUP

200g / 1½ cups blanched
  hazelnuts
2 tbsp coconut sugar
2 tbsp raw cacao powder
½ tsp maple syrup
½ tsp hazelnut oil
drop of vanilla extract
pinch of sea salt

Preheat the oven to 200°C / 400°F / gas mark 6.

Place the hazelnuts on a small baking tray (pan) and bake for 10 minutes to toast (keep an eye on them though so that they don't burn). Remove from the oven and set aside to cool.

Add the toasted, cooled hazelnuts to a food processor and blitz for about 3 minutes until they are broken down and have turned into a paste with their natural oils.

Add the remaining ingredients and blitz for another 2 minutes. Taste to check for flavour – you can add a pinch more sweetness if you like.

Transfer to a sterilized sealable jar and store at room temperature for up to 2 months.

Two Fruit Compotes

EACH MAKES 500G / 17½OZ

APPLE & PEAR

500g / 17½oz mixture of
  apples and pears, peeled,
  cored and roughly chopped
½ vanilla pod (bean)
40g / 2 tbsp agave syrup
200ml / ¾ cup water
small pinch of sea salt

FIG & GINGER

300g / 10½oz fresh figs,
  trimmed and quartered
20g / ¾oz fresh root ginger,
  peeled and grated
30g / 1½ tbsp honey
100ml / 7 tbsp water
small pinch of sea salt

Add all the ingredients to a medium saucepan, bring to the boil, then reduce the heat to low (covering with a lid for the apple and pear recipe), so that the fruit gently bubbles away as it breaks down. Stir occasionally to avoid the compote catching.

Let the compote simmer gently (Apple & Pear for 35–40 minutes; Fig & Ginger for 25 minutes), then remove from the heat and let cool completely. Store in the fridge for up to 5 days.

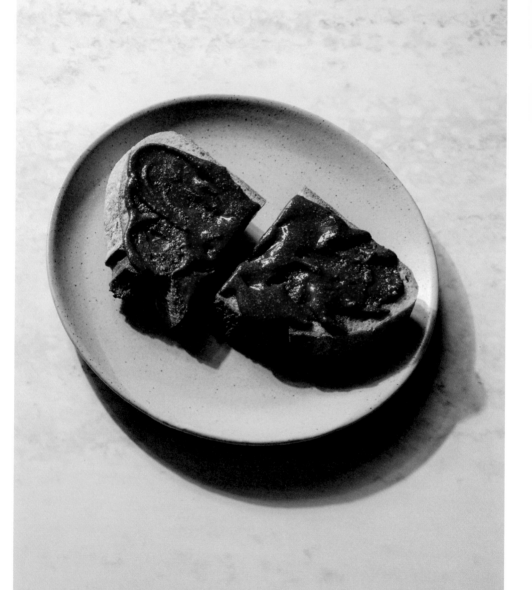

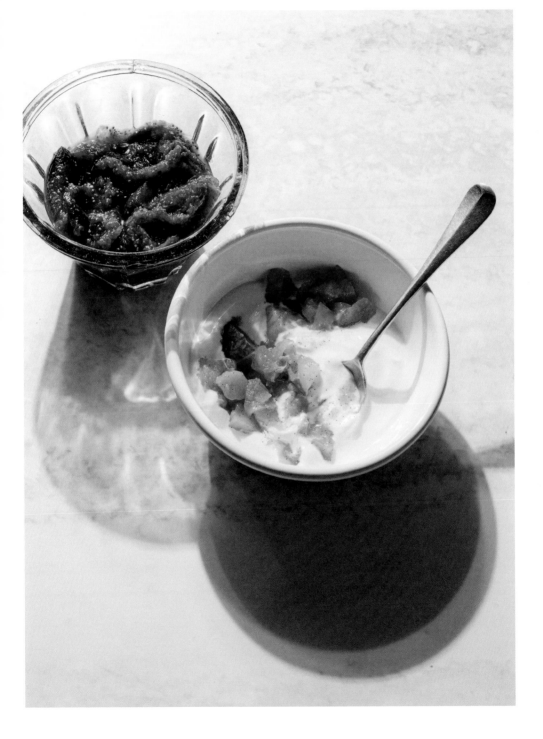

Energy Bites

MAKES 8 BITES

80g / ¾ cup porridge oats

80g / scant ⅓ cup peanut
  butter or almond butter

50g / 4 tbsp coconut oil,
  melted

30g / ¼ cup raisins

20g / 1 tbsp honey

40g / ½ cup desiccated (dried
  shredded) coconut

Add all the ingredients (reserving half the desiccated /
shredded coconut) to a saucepan and, on a low heat, stir
well to combine, just until the coconut oil and peanut
butter have loosened completely. Remove from the heat
and let cool for 5 minutes.

Sprinkle half the remaining coconut into the base of a
medium Tupperware box, then pile on the warm mixture,
flatten out and compress it with the back of a spoon.
Sprinkle the rest of the coconut evenly on top, let cool
completely, then seal with the lid and transfer to the fridge
to set overnight.

Once the slab has set, either remove the entire block and
slice up, or just cut out chunks as and when you like.

Store in the fridge for up to 5 days. You can also freeze it
for up to 1 month.

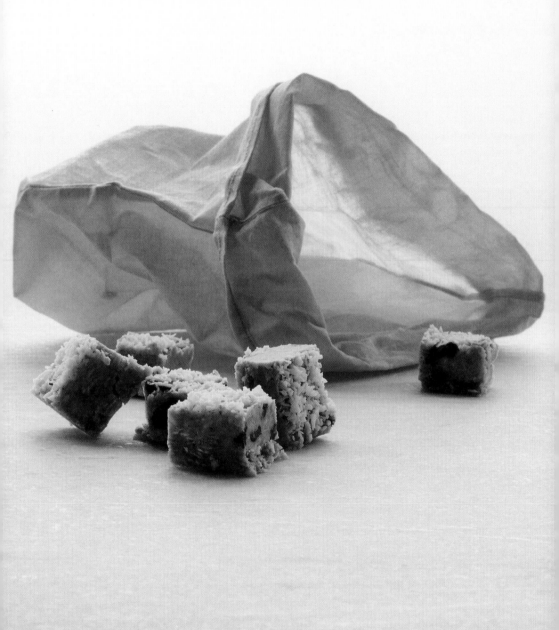

Banana &
Almond Pancakes

MAKES 12 PANCAKES

1 very ripe, or overripe,
  banana
1 egg
½ tsp vanilla extract
100g / ¾ cup wholemeal
  self-raising (self-rising)
  flour (or use white)
¼ tsp sea salt
about 150ml / ⅔ cup full-fat
  milk (or almond milk)
50g / ⅔ cup flaked (slivered)
  almonds, plus extra to serve
butter, for frying
yoghurt, blueberries and
  honey (optional), to serve

Add the banana, egg and vanilla to a medium bowl
and mash to break down the banana and combine
the ingredients.

In a large, separate bowl, add the flour and salt. Make
a well in the centre and add the egg/banana mixture
and half the milk. Whisk from the centre, working your
way to the edges and gradually incorporating the flour.
Once everything is combined, add more milk until you
have a thick, but sloppy consistency. Tip in the almonds
and fold through to combine.

Rest the batter in the fridge for 20 minutes.

Add a knob of butter to a large, non-stick frying pan
on a low heat. When very gently sizzling, add a generous
dessertspoon of batter to the pan, and repeat so you
have 2 or 3 pancakes on the go.

Cook gently for 2–4 minutes until the base is golden
and little air bubbles have risen to the surface, then flip
over and cook for another 1 minute or so. Transfer to a
plate and repeat with the remaining batter.

Serve with yoghurt, blueberries, extra almonds and a
small drizzle of honey, if you need it.

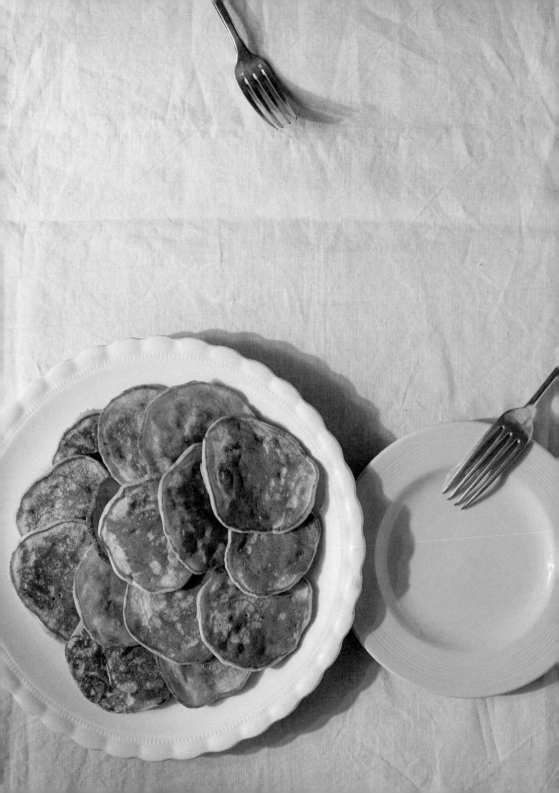

Hot Croissant Sarnies

SERVES 4

4 fresh croissants
2 bananas, sliced
Homemade Nutella (page 26)
almond butter
fresh berries (a mix)
whipped cream or yoghurt

Preheat the oven to 200°C / 400°F / gas mark 6.

Slice open the croissants like a sandwich and lay on a baking tray (pan) with the cut sides facing up. Transfer to the oven and warm up for 5 minutes.

Remove from the oven, transfer to plates and top one half with a selection of toppings, treating the open croissants like pancakes, then close to create sarnies. I like to have all the toppings out on the table so people can build their own.

(You can also do this with ham and cheese: lay the cheese on one half of the open croissants, warm in the oven for 5 minutes to melt the cheese, then add the ham and close to make sarnies.)

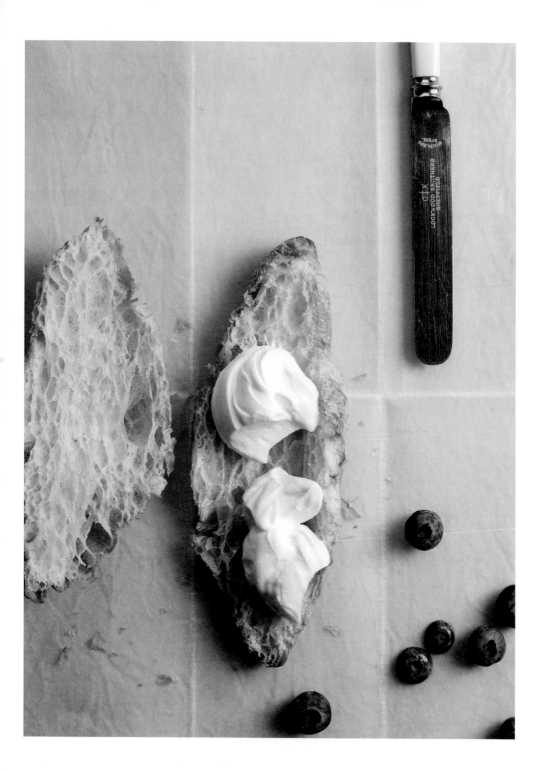

Cornbread with Crispy Smoked Bacon, Crème Fraîche & Pesto

Preheat the oven to 230°C / 450°F / gas mark 8.

SERVES 4

150g / 1 cup cornmeal
1 tsp baking powder
1 tsp coconut sugar, sifted
1 tsp sea salt
¼ tsp dried chilli flakes
180ml / ¾ cup buttermilk
1 egg, beaten
30g / 2 tbsp salted butter
drizzle of olive oil
8 slices of smoked streaky
  bacon
4 tbsp crème fraîche (or sour
  cream)
4 tbsp fresh pesto
1 red chilli, finely sliced

Add the cornmeal, baking powder, sugar, salt and chilli flakes to a large mixing bowl and stir to combine.

In a smaller bowl, mix the buttermilk and egg, beating with a fork to combine.

Add 20g / 1½ tbsp of the butter to a small ovenproof frying pan (about 20cm / 8in diameter) and melt, then let it turn to a brown butter. Remove from the heat, stir the butter to cool slightly, then gradually pour the brown butter into the wet ingredients, whisking constantly (to avoid cooking the eggs), then add this to the dry ingredients and fold to create a batter.

Heat the remaining butter in the same frying pan on a medium heat and, once sizzling, reduce the heat slightly to low–medium and add the batter. Spread out to the edges, then gently and evenly pat down with a spatula, frying for 2–3 minutes (don't stir) to form a nice golden crust on the base. Transfer to the top shelf of the oven and bake for 15–20 minutes.

Use a skewer to check that it's cooked through, then transfer the hot pan to a cooling rack and let cool completely before turning the cornbread out onto a plate. Wipe out the pan, then heat a small drizzle of oil in the pan on a medium–high heat. Once hot, add the bacon and fry for 8–10 minutes until crispy.

Quarter the cornbread, plate up and top with a dollop of crème fraîche, pesto, crispy bacon and some fresh chilli.

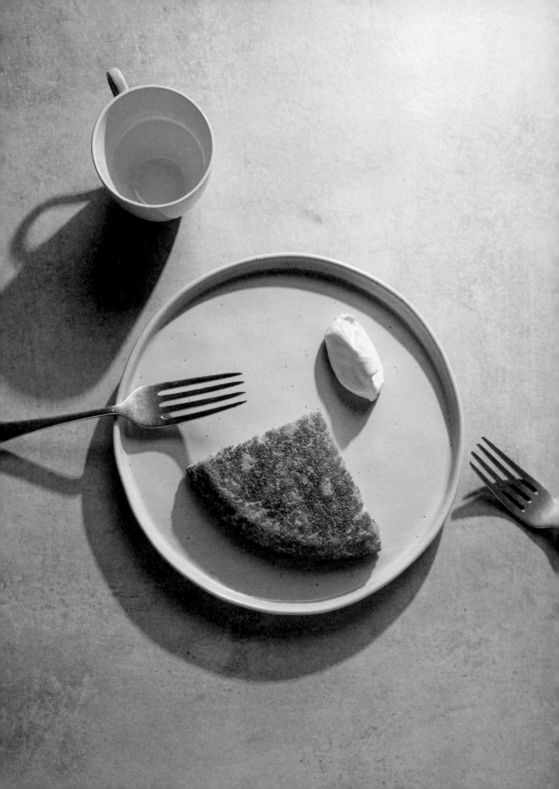

Seed & Parmesan Bread

MAKES 1 LOAF

(12–15 THIN SLICES)

oil, for greasing

4 eggs

500g / 17½oz seeds
  (use a mix of pumpkin
  seeds, chia seeds, sunflower
  seeds, pine nuts)

60g / 2oz Parmesan, finely
  grated

1 tsp sea salt

1 tbsp finely chopped fresh
  parsley

Preheat the oven to 220°C / 425°F / gas mark 7.

Grease a non-stick 24 x 14cm / 9½ x 5½in loaf tin (pan) and line with parchment paper.

Add the eggs to a large mixing bowl and beat with a fork to break up. Add the remaining ingredients to the bowl and mix with the fork very well to combine.

Pile the bread mixture into the lined tin, transfer to the middle shelf of the oven and bake for 40 minutes.

Transfer to a cooling rack and let cool in the tin for 5 minutes, then remove from the tin and allow to cool completely.

It is best served like toast. Store in the fridge for up to 5 days, or slice up and freeze for up to 1 month.

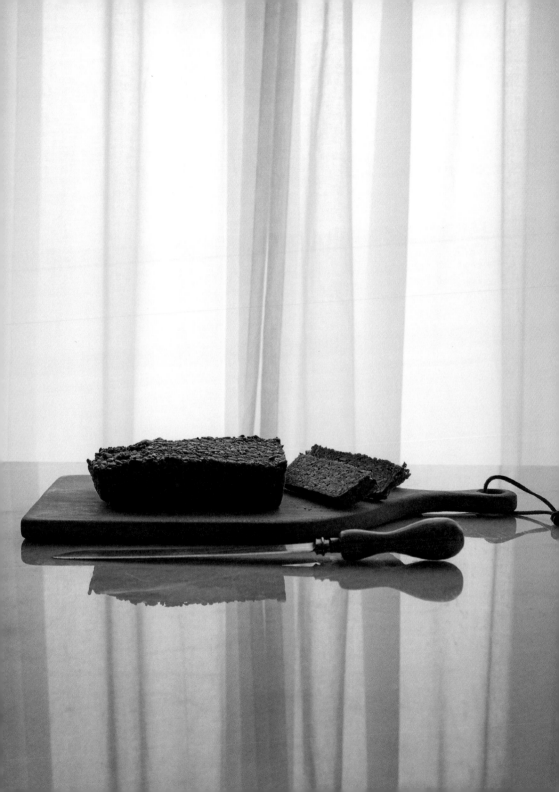

Berry Blossom Lassi

\\\\\\\\\\\\\\\\\\\\\\\\\\\\\\\\\\

SERVES 1

40g / 1½oz raspberries
200g / 7oz strawberries
100g / scant ½ cup plain
  yoghurt
¼ tsp orange blossom water
pinch of ground cardamom
handful of ice, to serve

Add all the ingredients to a Nutribullet or high-powered blender and blitz until very smooth.

Serve over ice.

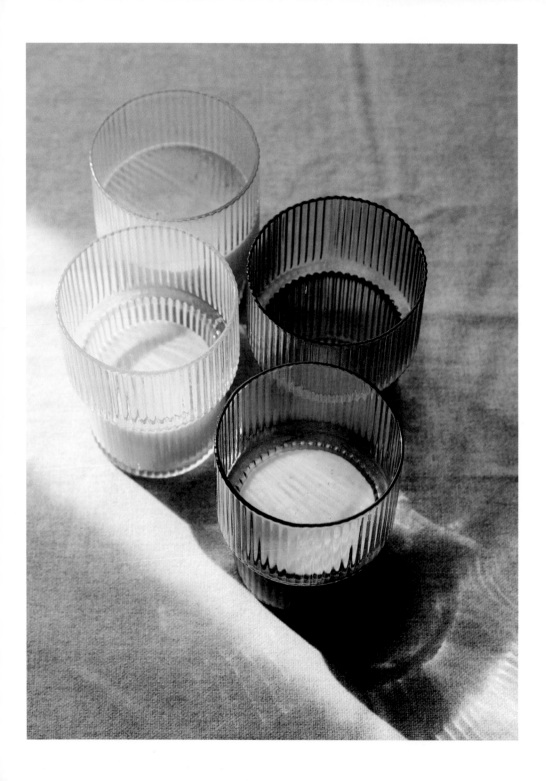

Brie & Grape Toasties

SERVES 4

6 tbsp mayonnaise

8 slices of bread (your choice)

160g / 5¾oz seedless red grapes, halved

3 tbsp Dijon mustard

4 spring onions (scallions), finely sliced

140g / 5oz Brie, thinly sliced

butter and olive oil, for frying

Spread the mayonnaise on one side of each slice of bread (like you would with butter).

Add the grapes, mustard and spring onions (scallions) to a bowl and mix very well to coat and combine.

Turn the mayo sides of 4 of the bread slices onto their backs (so the bare side is facing up). Layer on the Brie, then top with the grape, onion and mustard mixture. Place the second slice of bread on top, with the mayo side on the outside, to give you 4 sandwiches.

Heat a knob of butter and a small drizzle of olive oil in a large, non-stick frying pan on a low heat and add one (or two, depending on the size of your pan) toastie(s) to the pan. Fry on one side for 3–5 minutes, or until the base is golden brown and the Brie is starting to melt. Carefully turn and fry on the other side until you have a second golden-brown side and the Brie is gloriously gooey.

Transfer to a plate and cook the remaining toasties.

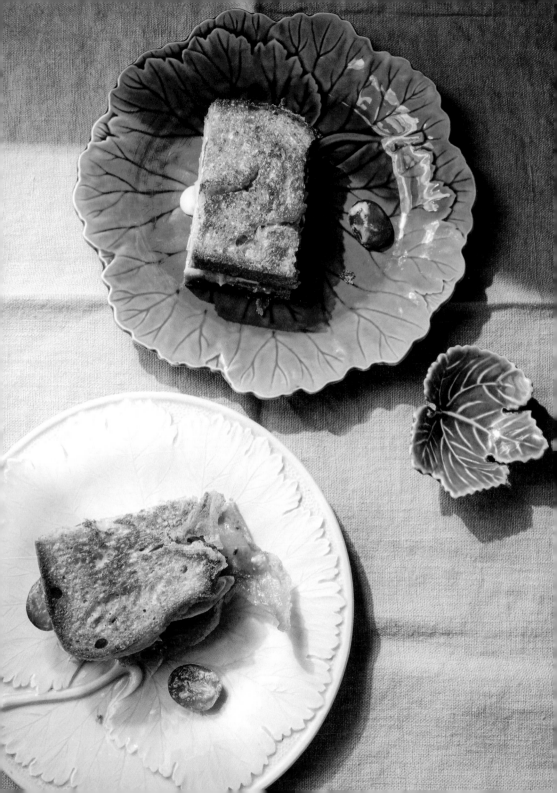

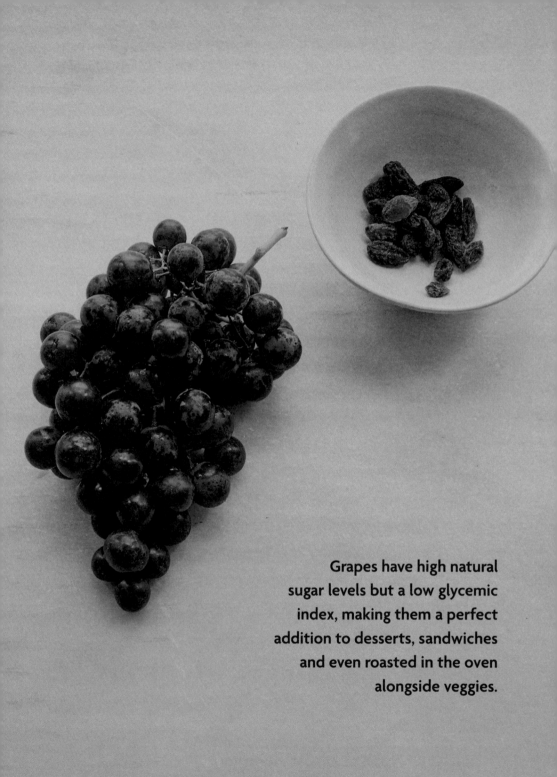

Grapes have high natural sugar levels but a low glycemic index, making them a perfect addition to desserts, sandwiches and even roasted in the oven alongside veggies.

Dried fruit has naturally high sugar levels so can be used in small amounts to sweeten jams, chutneys, puds and savoury dishes.

Cheese & Pickle Baguettes

\\\\\\\\\\\\\\\\\\\\\\\\\\\\\\\\\\\\

SERVES 4

1 large baguette, halved
  lengthways
200g / 7oz Cheddar, sliced
12 Baby Gem lettuce leaves
4 vine tomatoes, sliced
4 tbsp mayonnaise
8 slices of Parma ham

PICKLE

drizzle of olive oil
2 apples, grated
1 clove garlic, grated
60g / 2oz cornichons, finely
  sliced
pinch of dried chilli flakes
4 tbsp apple cider vinegar
4 tbsp coconut sugar
4 tbsp water
30g / ⅓ cup sultanas (golden
  raisins)
pinch of sea salt

To make the pickle, add the oil to a small saucepan on a medium heat and, once hot, add the apple, garlic and cornichons. Fry gently for 5 minutes, then add the rest of the pickle ingredients. Bring to the boil, then reduce the heat and let bubble for 10 minutes.

Build the baguettes with the filling ingredients, and spoon in the warm pickle. Serve with a beer.

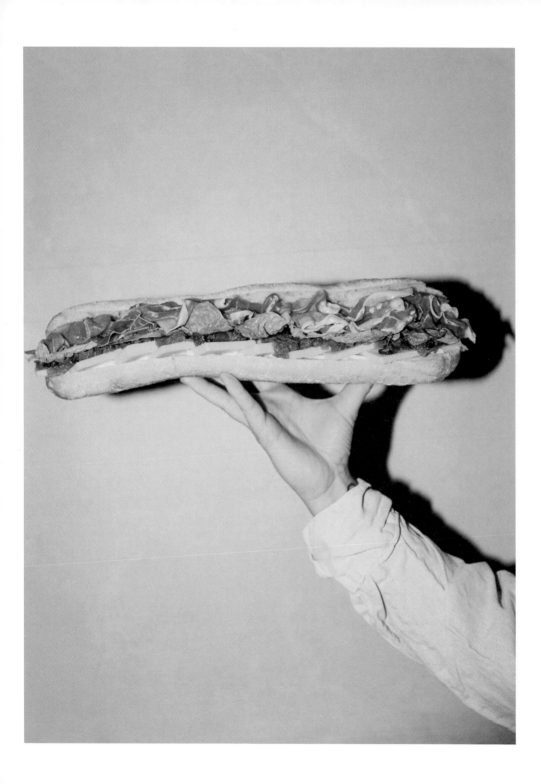

Fancy a fruity drink but trying to avoid fizzy pop and squash that are packed with refined sugar?

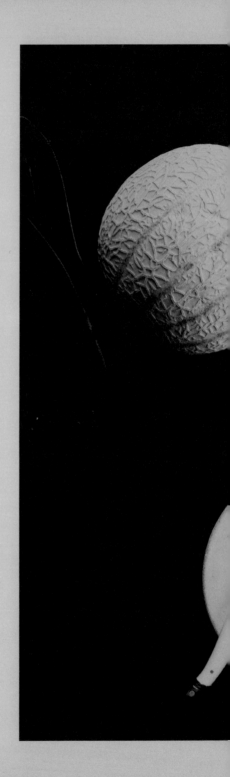

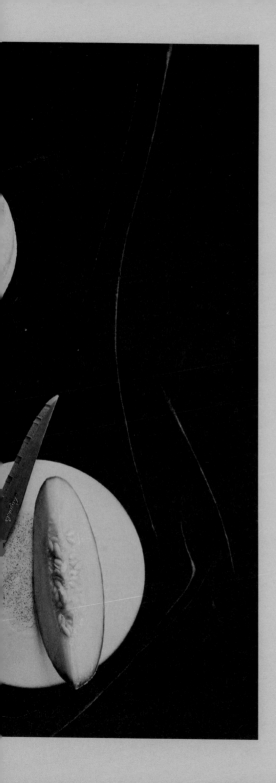

Instead, whip up a batch of cordial or infused water using citrus and fragrant fruits such as melon, apricots or peaches for a thirst-quenching hit that everyone will love.

Apricot Cordial

MAKES 350ML / 1½ CUPS

150g / 1 cup dried apricots

200ml / ¾ cup boiling water

3 tbsp honey

300ml / 1¼ cups cold water

juice of 1 lemon, or to taste

fizzy water, fresh mint and
   lemon slices, to serve

Add the apricots to a large Nutribullet cup (or the jug of a high-powered blender), pour in the boiling water to cover and leave to soak for 30 minutes.

Add the honey and blitz until very, very smooth.

Transfer to a saucepan, add the cold water and bring up to the boil. Reduce the heat and let bubble for 5 minutes.

Remove from the heat, pass through a sieve (strainer) and leave to cool. Add lemon juice to taste, then transfer the cordial to the fridge and store for up to 2 weeks.

Serve with fizzy water, fresh mint and lemon slices.

Watermelon & Lime Pitcher

SERVES 4

1kg / 2lb 3oz watermelon
  flesh
juice of 2 limes, plus extra
  if needed
10g / ⅓oz mint, leaves only
100ml / 7 tbsp water
ice, to serve

Place a serving jug (pitcher) in the freezer while you prepare the drink.

Add all the ingredients except the ice to a blender and blitz until very smooth. Taste and add more lime juice if needed.

Transfer to the chilled serving jug along with plenty of ice, and serve immediately.

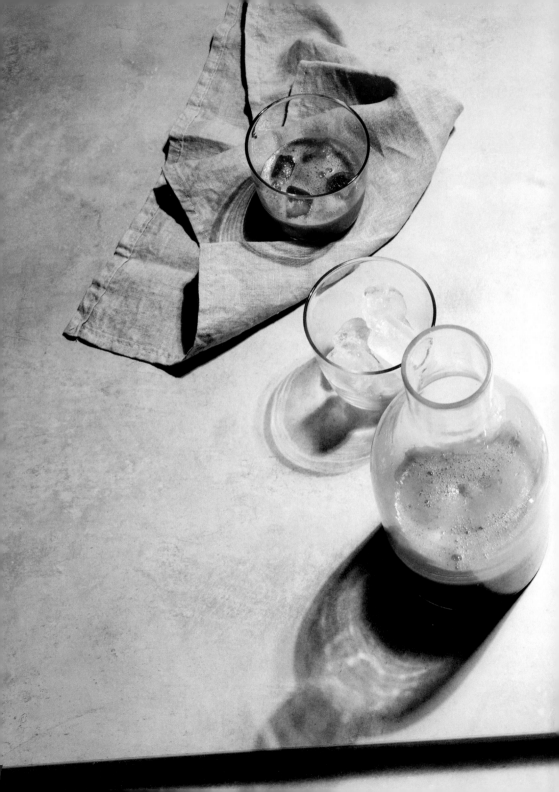

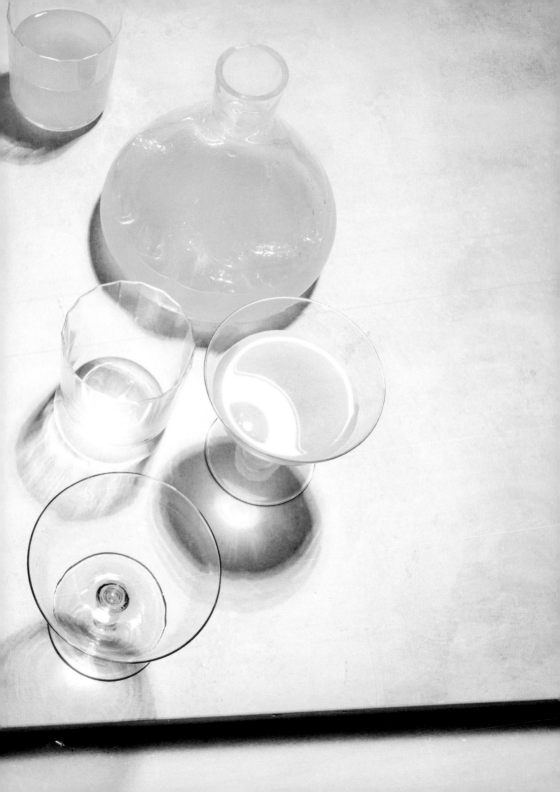

Strawberry, Basil & Goat's Cheese Salad

SERVES 4 AS A STARTER OR SIDE

50g / 1¾oz fresh basil leaves

3 tbsp olive oil

1 tsp apple cider vinegar

1 clove garlic, peeled

80g / ⅔ cup pine nuts, toasted

pinch of sea salt

¼ tsp cracked black pepper

squeeze of lemon juice

100g / 2 cups watercress

150g / 1½ cups strawberries, hulled and quartered lengthways, or halved if small

150g / 5¼oz soft goat's cheese

20g / ¾oz mixed seeds

Add the basil to a food processor with the oil, vinegar, garlic, 50g / generous ⅓ cup of the pine nuts, salt and pepper and whizz until smooth. Taste, and add a squeeze of lemon juice and more seasoning if needed.

Add the watercress to a salad bowl along with the strawberries and remaining pine nuts, then scoop off chunks of soft goat's cheese and add to the salad. Drizzle over half the basil dressing and gently toss.

Serve immediately, with an extra drizzle of the basil dressing around the plate.

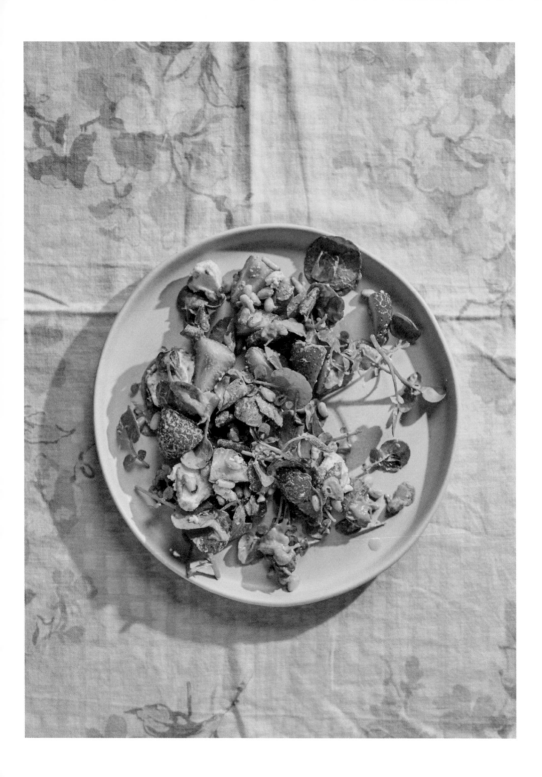

Griddled Pineapple Salad

SERVES 4

1 pineapple
drizzle of rapeseed
　(canola) oil
10g / ⅓oz fresh mint
15g / ½oz fresh coriander
　(cilantro)
60g / 2oz rocket (arugula)
30g / 1oz crispy onions
1 red chilli, finely sliced
1 lime, zested then cut into
　wedges
sea salt and freshly ground
　black pepper
extra virgin olive oil, to serve

Heat a griddle pan on a medium heat.

Cut off the top of the pineapple and trim the base. Stand the pineapple up and carefully slice off the peel, working down the sides, then cut the flesh into wedges, removing the tough core.

Drizzle the wedges with a little rapeseed oil and season with salt and pepper, like a steak.

Once the griddle pan is really hot, add the pineapple wedges and cook for 3–4 minutes on each side until nicely charred.

Meanwhile, pick the mint leaves from the stems and add to a large, shallow dish with the coriander (cilantro) stems and rocket (arugula) and toss to combine. Top with the griddled pineapple, then sprinkle over the crispy onions, chilli and lime zest.

Drizzle a bit of extra virgin olive oil over the whole thing and serve immediately, with the lime wedges for squeezing.

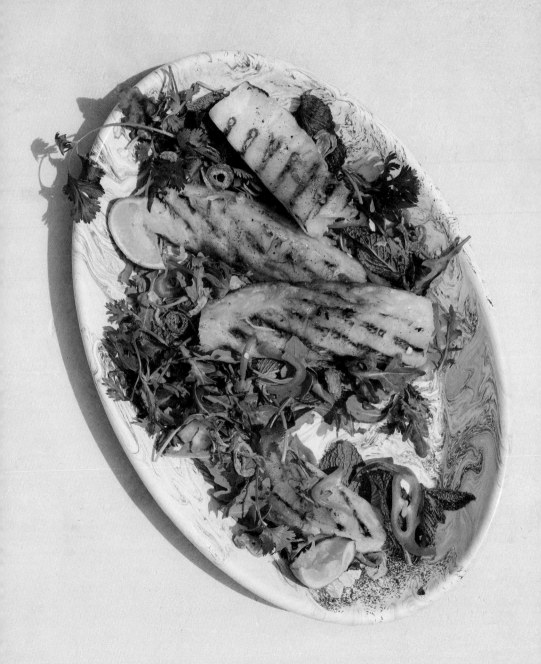

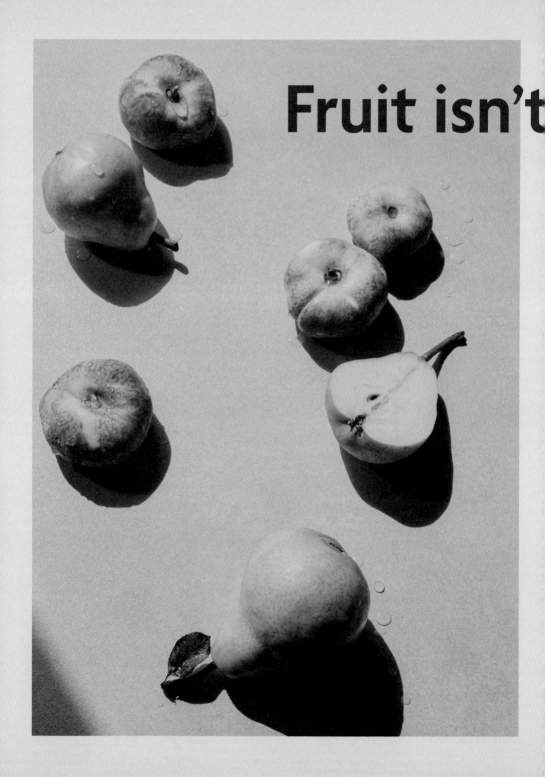

Fruit isn't

ust for dessert

– try pears, peaches
and pineapple griddled
in salads, or added to
tray bakes, and berries
like strawberries and
raspberries paired with
soft cheeses, for sweet
and sour flavour combos
that pack a punch.

Summer Rolls with Sweet Chilli Sauce

SERVES 4 AS A STARTER

100g / 3½oz vermicelli rice
noodles

1 carrot, peeled and cut into
long matchsticks

⅓ cucumber, cut into long
matchsticks

1 red (bell) pepper,
deseeded and cut into long
matchsticks

10g / ⅓oz fresh mint, leaves
picked

10g / ⅓oz coriander (cilantro)
sprigs

100g / 3½oz cooked peeled
prawns (shrimp)

drizzle of rice vinegar

pinch of sea salt

4–6 rice paper wraps,
20cm / 8in diameter

SWEET CHILLI GARLIC SAUCE

1 fresh red chilli, finely
chopped (seeds in)

1 clove garlic, finely chopped

pinch of dried chilli flakes

4 tbsp water

4 tbsp white wine vinegar

1 tsp fish sauce

2 tsp palm sugar

2 tbsp agave

pinch of sea salt

Add all the ingredients for the sweet chilli garlic sauce
to a small pan, bring to a boil and bubble vigorously for
3 minutes. Take off the heat and leave to cool.

Cook the rice noodles according to the packet
instructions, drain and run cold water through them to
cool; drain fully.

Lay out the noodles, veg sticks, herbs and prawns
(shrimp) in separate piles and drizzle a very small amount
of rice vinegar over the veg. Add a pinch of sea salt, to
gently season it all.

Soak the rice paper wraps according to the packet
instructions (about 5 seconds in warm–hot water), then
lay one out on a chopping board. Place some filling
ingredients down the middle, leaving a generous clear
space either end. Start with the prawns and mint, then the
veg, then the noodles and finally the coriander (cilantro).

Fold over half of the clear wrap on top of the filling, as
you would for a burrito, then bring over each short end on
top, and roll the folded section over itself to complete and
seal the roll. Transfer to a plate, repeat with the remaining
ingredients and serve with the sweet chilli garlic sauce.

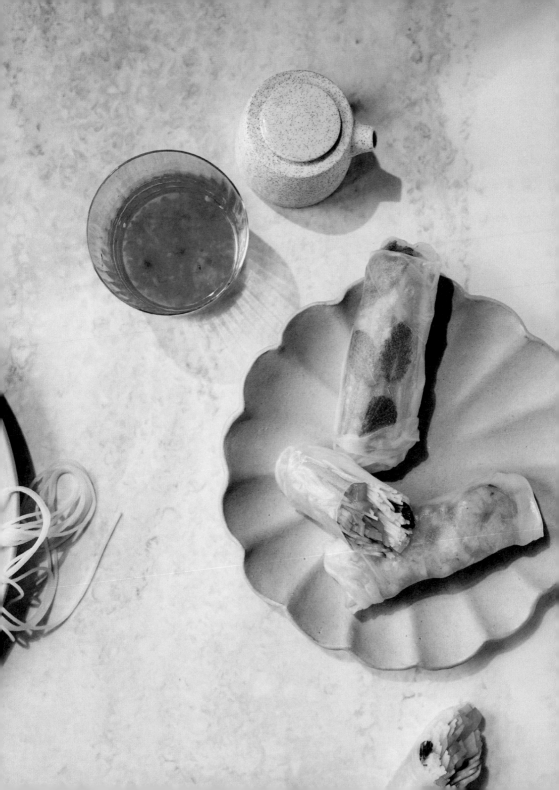

Honey Roasted Nuts

SERVES 4 AS A SNACK

250g / 8¾oz mixed nuts

2 tbsp olive oil

1 tbsp polenta

2 tbsp runny honey

1 tsp smoked paprika

½ tsp ground cumin

½ tsp sea salt

1 tsp butter, melted

3 sprigs of fresh rosemary

Preheat the oven to 190°C / 375°F / gas mark 5.

Add all the ingredients to a mixing bowl and toss very well to combine and coat.

Spread the coated nuts evenly out on a large non-stick baking tray (pan), making sure you get all the marinade out of the bowl – use a silicone spatula to scrape it all out.

Bake on the middle shelf of the oven for 20 minutes, turning the nuts halfway through.

Remove from the oven and let cool completely, then transfer to an airtight container and store at room temperature for up to 5 days.

Coconut Magarita

SERVES 2

juice of 2 limes

5g / 1 tbsp desiccated (dried shredded) coconut, toasted

¼ tsp flaky sea salt

1 fresh jalapeño chilli

2 shots of tequila

2 tbsp triple sec

2 shots of coconut water

ice, to shake and serve

Put the lime juice into a bowl that has a wider circumference than that of the glasses you're serving the drinks in, then place the desiccated (shredded) coconut and sea salt on a small side plate and mix to combine.

Dip the rims of the glasses in the lime juice, then immediately in the coconut–salt mixture, then half-fill the glasses with ice.

Halve the chilli lengthways and add a half to each glass.

Add the lime juice, tequila, triple sec and coconut water along with a handful of ice to a cocktail shaker (or just a large sealable container, like a jar) and shake very well to mix.

Strain the cocktail into the glasses and serve immediately.

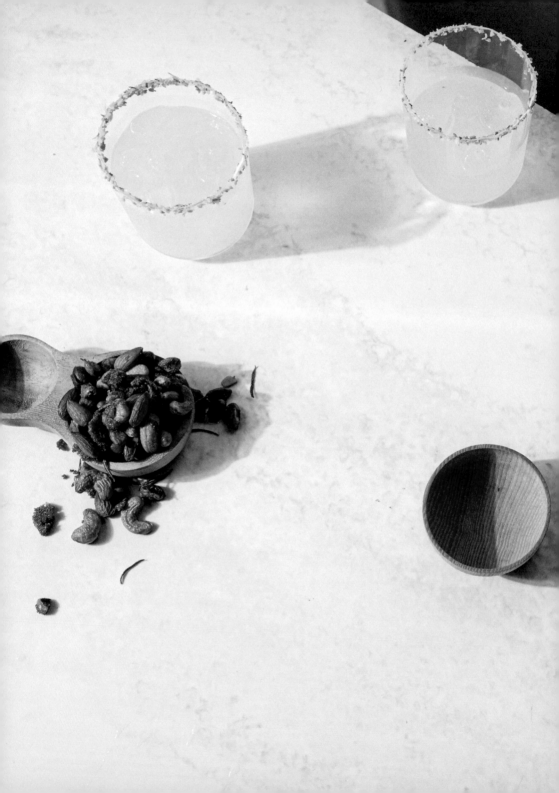

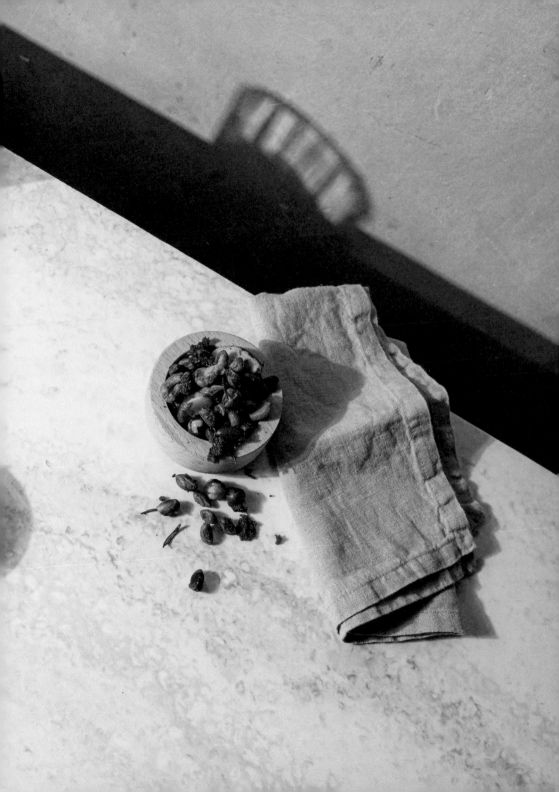

Coconuts are an amazing source of natural sweetness.

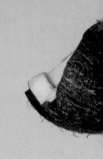

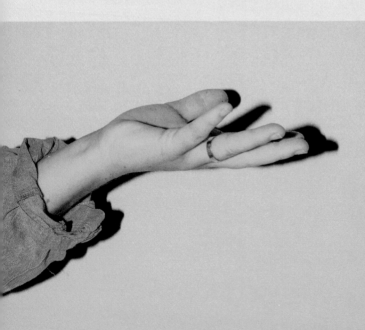

Experiment using coconut flesh, as well as its milk, water and sugar, and desiccated (shredded) coconut to add a creamy, sweet flavour to a range of different dishes.

Chicken Satay Wings & Smashed Cucumber

SERVES 4 AS A STARTER

800g / 1¾lb chicken wings

2 tbsp fish sauce

1 tbsp light soy sauce

juice of ½ lime

sea salt and freshly ground
   black pepper

SATAY SAUCE

40g / 1½oz fresh root ginger,
   peeled and grated

2 cloves garlic, grated

160g / ¾ cup smooth peanut
   butter

1 tbsp light soy sauce

2 tsp honey

200ml / ¾ cup coconut milk

BASHED CUCUMBER SALAD

300g / 10½oz cucumber

1 tbsp sesame oil

1 tbsp rice wine vinegar

1 tbsp sesame seeds (white,
   black or mixed)

¼ tsp dried chilli flakes

TO SERVE

1 red chilli, finely sliced

10g / ⅓oz fresh coriander
   (cilantro), torn

Preheat the oven to 200°C / 400°F / gas mark 6.

Add the chicken wings to a large mixing bowl with the
fish sauce, soy sauce, lime juice and some seasoning. Mix
well to coat the wings, then transfer to a baking tray (pan),
pouring any remaining marinade on top. Roast on the top
shelf of the oven for 30 minutes, basting halfway through.

Meanwhile, to make the satay sauce, heat a medium
saucepan and, once hot, add the ginger and garlic (no oil)
to the pan. Let gently sizzle for a minute, stirring almost
constantly to avoid burning, then add the peanut butter
and let that loosen for another minute, stirring often.
Next, add the soy sauce, honey and coconut milk and
bring to just below a simmer. The sauce may split if it is
on the heat for too long, so reduce the temperature to low
and cook very gently for 1 minute, whisking constantly
to combine, emulsify and smooth out. If the sauce splits,
just add a drop or two of cold water and whisk vigorously.
Remove the pan from the heat and set aside.

When the wings have been in the oven for 30 minutes,
dollop on one-third of the satay sauce (still on the baking
tray) and return to the oven for 10 minutes.

Roughly chop the cucumber into 3–4cm / 1¼–1½in
chunks, then bash them a bit, using a rolling pin or small
saucepan. Add them to a small serving dish along with the
remaining salad ingredients and toss to combine.

Serve the satay wings topped with the chilli and coriander
(cilantro), with the cucumber salad, and the remaining
sauce on the side.

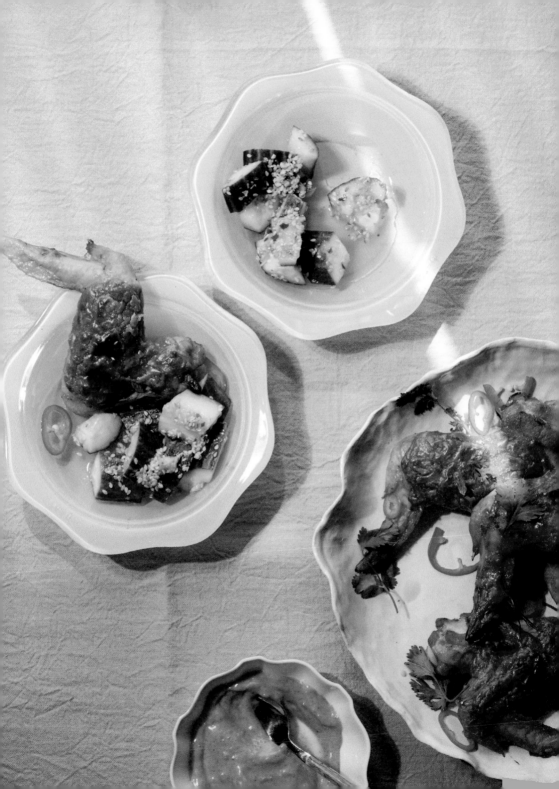

Duck Pancakes with Hoisin Sauce

///////////////////////////////

SERVES 4

4 confit duck legs (I use
  Gressingham Bistro)
1 cucumber
6 spring onions (scallions)
12–16 Chinese pancakes
  (shop-bought)

HOISIN SAUCE

½ tsp Chinese five spice
  powder
3 tbsp Doenjang soybean
  paste (Korean miso; found
  in Asian supermarkets or
  online)
5 Medjool dates, pitted
20g / 2 tbsp sultanas (golden
  raisins)
1 clove garlic, peeled
4 tbsp water
2 tbsp light soy sauce
1 tbsp red wine vinegar
1 tsp sesame oil
20g / generous 1 tbsp coconut
  sugar
pinch of sea salt

Preheat the oven to 200°C / 400°F / gas mark 6.

Place the duck legs on a baking tray (pan) and cook according to the packet instructions.

Cut the cucumber into matchsticks and do the same with the spring onions (scallions).

Add all the sauce ingredients to a food processor or blender and blitz until very smooth. The dates may take a while to break down, but persevere.

When the duck is roasted and ready, transfer to a board and shred, using 2 forks.

Serve the shredded duck with the pancakes, cucumber, spring onions and hoisin sauce.

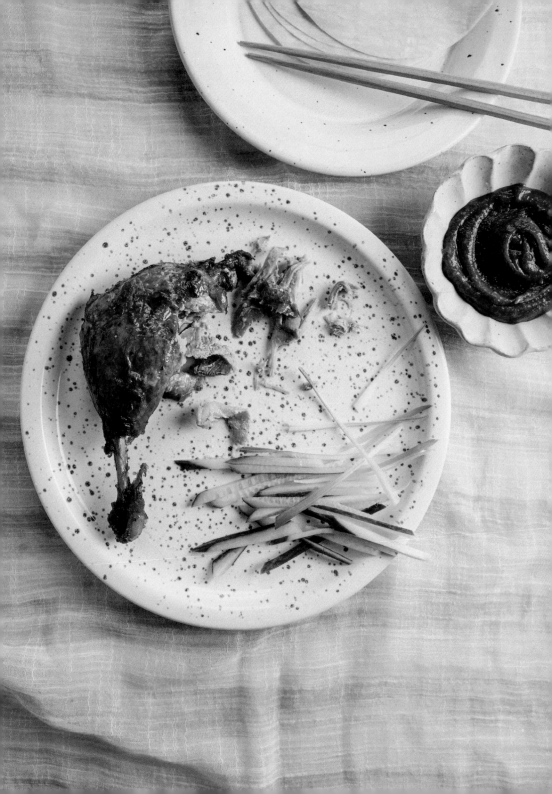

Roasted Squash Wedges

SERVES 4 AS A STARTER

1 tsp ground turmeric

1 tsp ground coriander

1 tsp pomegranate molasses

1 tbsp red wine vinegar

2 tbsp olive oil

2 cloves garlic, grated

1 butternut squash

2 spring onions (scallions),
 sliced

10g / ⅓oz coriander
 (cilantro), chopped

10g / ⅓oz dried cranberries,
 chopped

sea salt and freshly ground
 black pepper

TO SERVE

60g / 4 tbsp plain yoghurt

¼ tsp cracked black pepper

Preheat the oven to 220°C / 425°F / gas mark 7.

Add the ground turmeric and coriander, pomegranate molasses, vinegar, oil and garlic to a small bowl and mix to combine.

Quarter the butternut squash lengthways, remove the seeds and place the long wedges cut-side up in a roasting dish. Pour the spice mix over the butternut squash and then sprinkle over a pinch each of salt and pepper.

Place on the middle shelf of the oven and roast for about 1 hour until caramelized and tender.

Mix the spring onions (scallions), coriander (cilantro) and cranberries together.

Serve the squash on a sharing dish as a starter or a side, with a dollop of yoghurt on top, the cranberry mix and cracked black pepper.

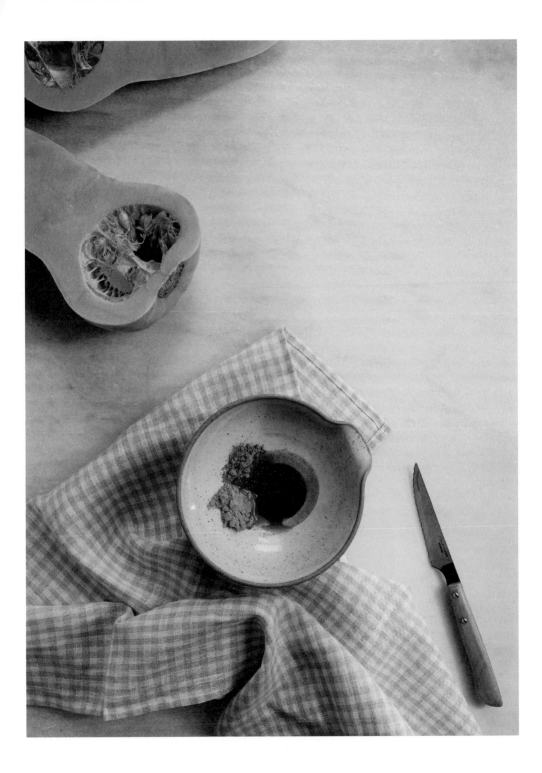

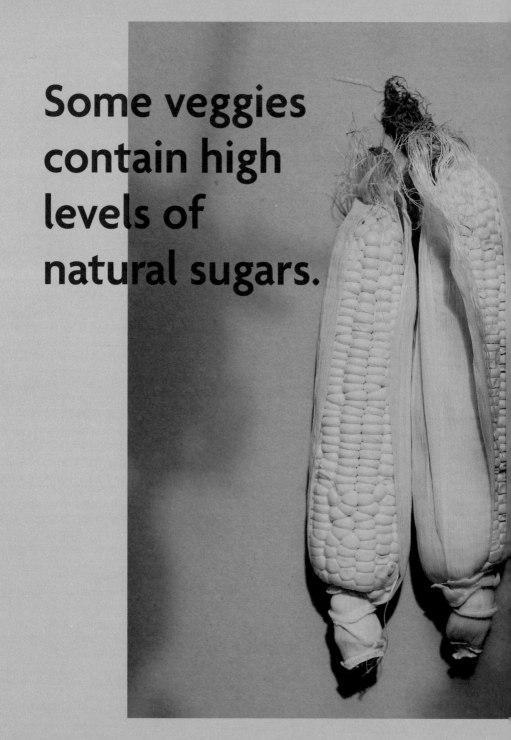

Some veggies contain high levels of natural sugars.

Try cooking with squash, pumpkin, sweet potato, swede, carrots, peas, sweetcorn or beetroot when you fancy a sweet but savoury supper.

Tangy Ketchup

MAKES ABOUT 400ML / 1²⁄₃ CUPS

generous drizzle of olive oil

2 onions, finely chopped

2 cloves garlic, finely
  chopped

½ tsp ground mixed spice

½ tsp ground cumin

1 tsp ground ginger

½ tsp ground coriander

1 bay leaf

1 tbsp tomato purée (paste)

1 tsp light soy sauce

50ml / 3½ tbsp date syrup

50ml / 3½ tbsp maple syrup

70ml / 4½ tbsp red wine
  vinegar

700g / 1½lb tomatoes
  (any sort; roughly chop
  larger than cherry size)

lemon juice, to taste
  (if needed)

sea salt and freshly ground
  black pepper

Heat the olive oil in a medium saucepan and, when hot, add the onions and sweat down for 10 minutes, stirring often to avoid catching.

Add the garlic, all the spices and ½ teaspoon salt and cook out for 1–2 minutes until very fragrant, then add the bay leaf, tomato purée (paste), soy sauce, date syrup, maple syrup, vinegar and tomatoes.

Bring to the boil, cover with a lid, reduce the heat to a gentle simmer and let bubble away for 20 minutes, stirring occasionally. Remove the lid and let simmer for another 30 minutes, stirring more often. You'll need to stand over the sauce for the last 10 minutes as it will have reduced down a lot and could be prone to catching.

Remove and discard the bay leaf, then transfer the mixture to a food processor and blend until very smooth; taste to check for seasoning and add more salt and pepper, and lemon juice, if you like (be aware that flavours will dull once cool). Leave to cool and store in a clean jar in the fridge for up to 1 month.

Mango Chutney

SERVES 4 AS A SNACK OR SIDE

1 mango

1 tsp coconut oil

1 shallot, finely chopped

2 cloves garlic, finely
  chopped

20g / ¾oz fresh root ginger,
  peeled and finely chopped

1 red chilli, trimmed,
  deseeded and finely diced

3 cardamom pods, bashed

2 cloves

1 star anise

¼ tsp nigella seeds

¼ tsp sea salt

½ tsp cornflour (cornstarch)

2 tbsp agave

1 tbsp apple cider vinegar

90ml / 6 tbsp water

Peel the mango and cut the flesh off from around the
stone (pit). You should have about 230g / 8oz flesh.
Cut into large chunks – it will break down in the pan,
so you want them big.

Heat the coconut oil in a medium saucepan on a
medium heat and, once hot, add the shallot. Let sweat
for 5 minutes until softening, then add the garlic, ginger,
chilli, cardamom, cloves, star anise, nigella seeds and
salt. Fry for another minute, stirring often, then add the
cornflour (cornstarch) and mix to combine.

Next add the agave, vinegar and water to the pan. Bring to
the boil, bubble for 2 minutes, then add the mango. Cover
with a lid and let simmer and break down for 10 minutes.

Remove from the heat, leave to cool, then transfer to
a clean, sterilized jar and store in the fridge for up to
3 months. Serve with poppadoms.

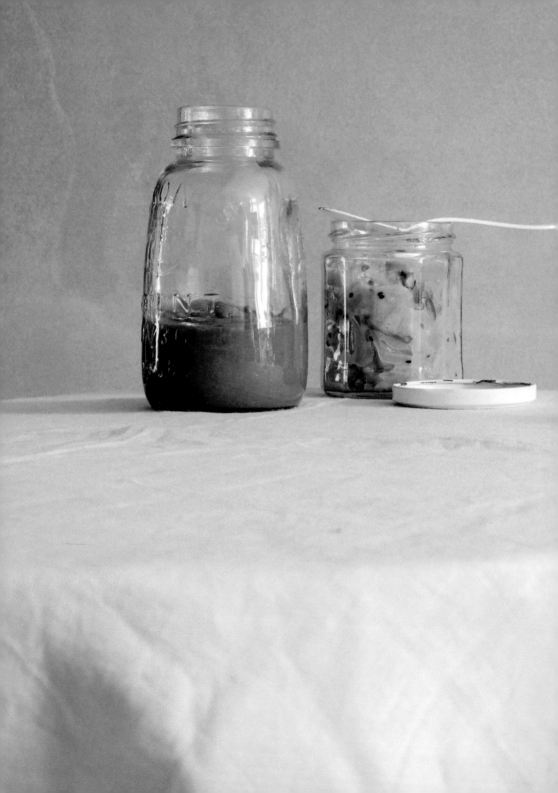

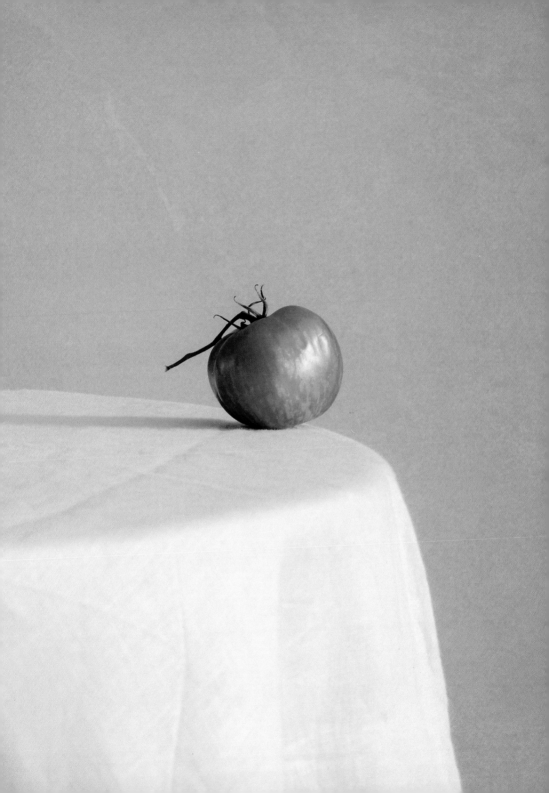

Be careful with sauces, condiments and flavourings – lots of them have refined sugars hidden within. Be sure to always check the label.

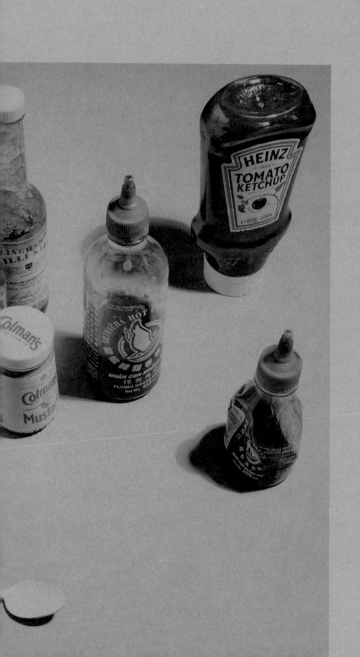

Spare Ribs

SERVES 2

3 tbsp dark soy sauce

2 tbsp ginger paste

2 cinnamon sticks

1 tbsp ground coriander

2 tbsp pomegranate molasses

1 tbsp olive oil

200ml / ¾ cup apple juice

650g / 1lb 7oz pork ribs,
  separated

sea salt and freshly ground
  black pepper

Add the soy sauce, ginger, cinnamon, ground coriander, pomegranate molasses, olive oil and apple juice to a roasting tin and mix well to combine. Add the ribs to the tin and coat them in the marinade, then cover with foil, transfer to the fridge and leave overnight.

Remove the ribs from the fridge and set aside at room temperature. Preheat the oven to 160°C / 320°F / gas mark 3.

Season the ribs very well with salt and pepper, seal the roasting tin with the foil and cook in the oven for 4 hours, basting every hour.

Remove the ribs and, while they sit for 5 minutes, transfer the marinade liquid in the roasting tin to a small saucepan, removing the cinnamon sticks, and bring to a boil. Reduce the sauce on a rapid boil for about 3–5 minutes until it is thick and silky.

Transfer the ribs to a chopping board or dish and pour over the reduced sauce. Serve with slaw (and baked potatoes, if you like).

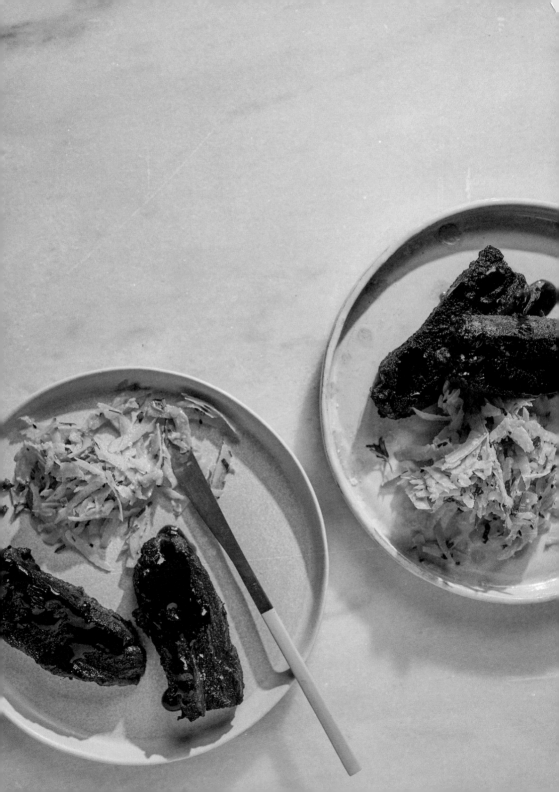

Sweet & Sour Chicken

SERVES 4

5 tbsp light soy sauce

5 tbsp date syrup

3 tbsp honey

7 tbsp rice wine vinegar

600g / 1lb 5oz chicken mini fillets

2 tbsp cornflour (cornstarch)

2 tbsp rapeseed (canola) oil, plus extra if needed for the veg

1 white onion, finely sliced

1 red (bell) pepper, deseeded and finely sliced

3 large cloves garlic, finely sliced

40g / 1½oz fresh root ginger, peeled and cut into matchsticks

1 x 400g / 14oz can pineapple chunks in juice, drained (260g / 9¼oz drained weight)

sea salt and freshly ground black pepper

TO SERVE

cooked rice

20g / ¾oz fresh coriander (cilantro)

1 lime, quartered

Add the soy sauce, date syrup, honey, vinegar and a pinch of seasoning to a bowl and mix to combine, then set aside.

Put the chicken in a large mixing bowl with a good pinch of seasoning and the cornflour (cornstarch). Toss well to coat the chicken in the seasoned cornflour.

Heat the oil in a large, non-stick frying pan on a high heat and, once hot, add the chicken and brown all over for 5–7 minutes. Transfer the browned chicken to a plate and put the pan back on a medium heat. Add the onion and (bell) pepper, with a fresh drizzle of oil if you need it.

Fry for 5 minutes until softening and beginning to colour, then add the garlic, ginger and pineapple and fry for 3 minutes. Add the chicken back into the pan, along with the soy sauce mixture.

Bring to the boil and let simmer for 7–10 minutes, or until the sauce is a coating consistency and the chicken is cooked through (check there is no pink in the middle). Remove from the heat and serve at once on top of rice, with coriander (cilantro) and lime wedges.

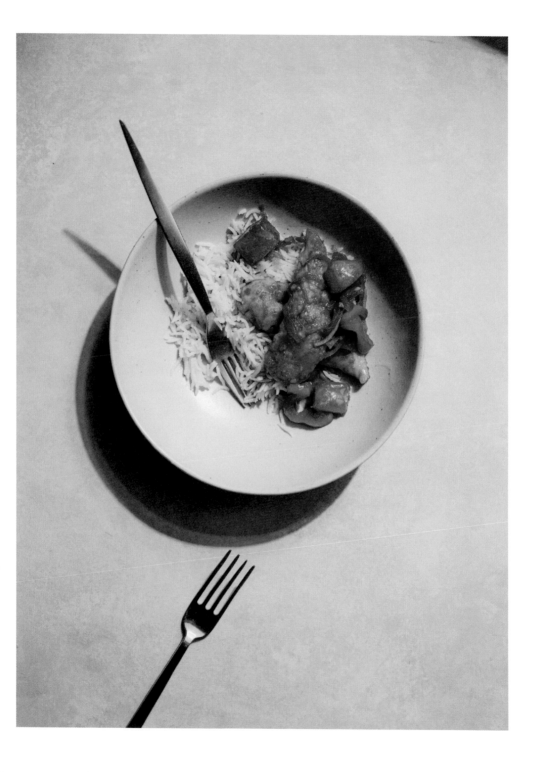

Pineapple & Rum Cocktail

SERVES 4

400g / 14oz fresh pineapple
  flesh, roughly chopped
juice of ½ lemon
4 shots of dark rum
handful of ice cubes
prosecco

Add the pineapple, lemon juice and rum to a NutriBullet or high-powered blender and blitz. Strain through a sieve into glasses filled with ice.

Top up with prosecco and serve immediately.

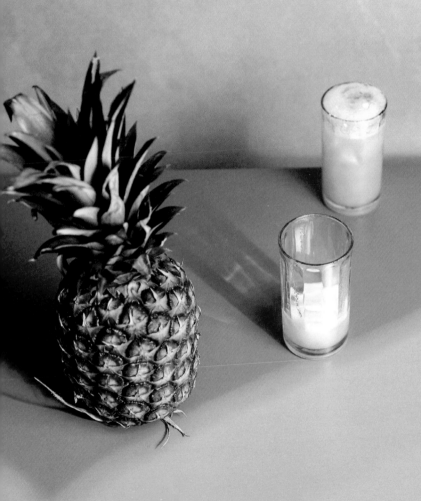

Baked BBQ Bananas

SERVES 4

4 ripe bananas

50g / 1¾oz nuts (cashews, walnuts, hazelnuts, peanuts or a mixture)

4–6 tbsp nut butter of your choice

10g / 2 tbsp desiccated (dried shredded) coconut

double (heavy) cream, to serve (optional)

Preheat the BBQ (grill), or the oven to 220°C / 425°F / gas mark 7.

Lay each whole (skin-on) banana on a large piece of foil. Cut a slit down the centre and length of the banana, cutting through the skin and flesh but not all the way to the base.

Fill each banana cavity with the nuts, nut butter and desiccated (shredded) coconut, then wrap the foil around the banana to seal each parcel.

If you are cooking on the BBQ, the parcels can go straight onto the grill; if you're using an oven, place the parcels on a baking tray (pan).

Cook for 20 minutes, then remove from the heat and let sit for a minute before handling.

Open the parcels and top the baked, stuffed and oozy bananas with a slosh of cream, if you like.

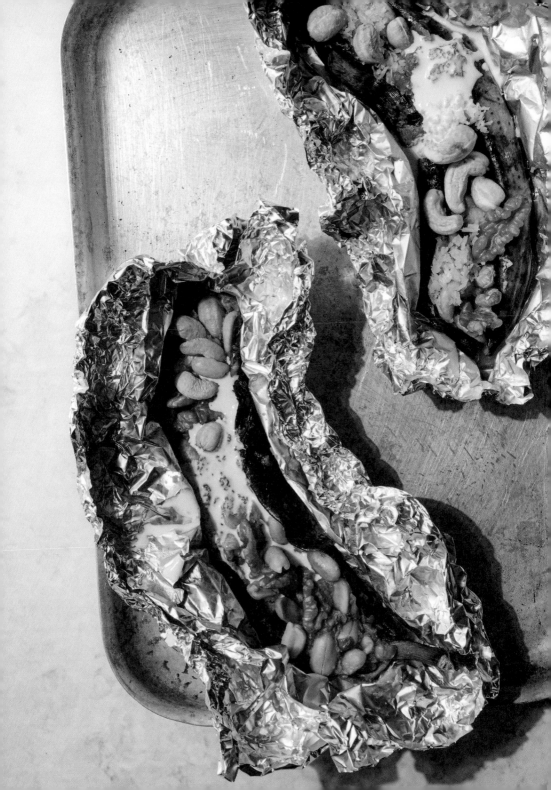

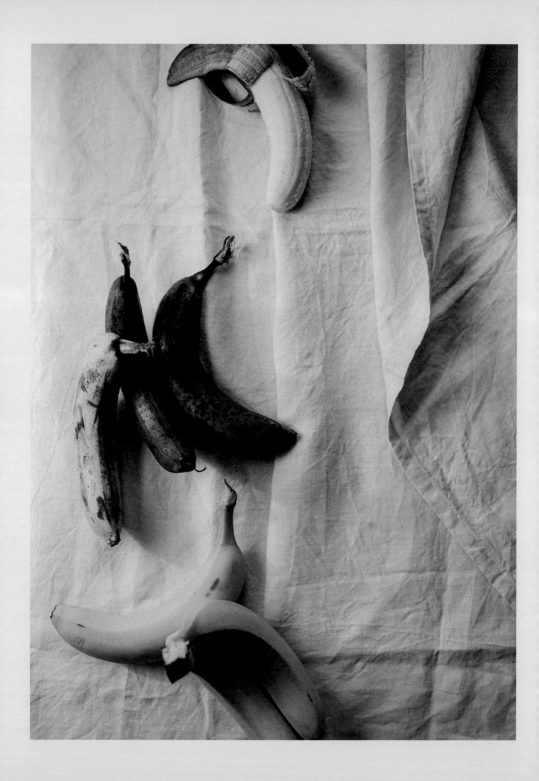

The browner bananas get, the sweeter they become.

Bear this is mind when using in desserts.

Chocolate Banana 'Ice Cream'

SERVES 2

3 tbsp cocoa powder

3 tbsp boiling water

4 overripe bananas, peeled,
   roughly chopped and frozen

1 tbsp almond butter

1 tbsp full-fat milk

a little 100% raw cacao
   chocolate, to serve
   (optional)

Add the cocoa powder and boiling water to a small bowl and mix well to make a paste.

Place the frozen banana pieces in a NutriBullet or high-powered food processor with the cocoa paste, almond butter and milk and blitz until smooth.

Either serve immediately or freeze for up to 1 month. It's best to re-blitz (with a small splash of milk) before serving, to smoothen the texture out again.

Serve with a little chocolate grated over the top, if you like.

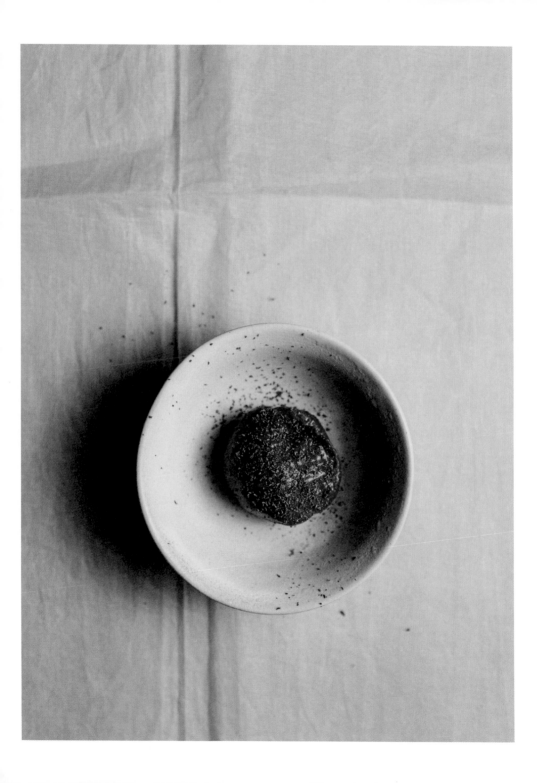

Coconut Doughnuts

MAKES 8 DOUGHNUTS

200g / scant 1½ cups strong
white bread flour
7g / ¼oz fast-action dried
yeast
20g / 2 tbsp coconut sugar,
sifted
¼ tsp sea salt
110g / 3½oz coconut milk
20g / 1½ tbsp salted butter
1 egg, beaten
1.5l / 6½ cups vegetable oil,
plus extra for greasing

GLAZE & TO FINISH

220ml / scant 1 cup coconut
milk
120g / ½ cup cream cheese
50g / ¼ cup coconut sugar,
sifted
zest and juice of 1 lime
30g / 5 tbsp desiccated (dried
shredded) coconut, toasted
(optional)

Add the dry ingredients to a stand mixer bowl, and mix to combine.

Melt and loosen the coconut milk and butter in a small saucepan. You want the mixture warm, but not hot, when it goes into the bowl.

Make a well in the dry ingredients, add the coconut milk and butter mixture to the well, and begin to gradually combine. Once the warm, wet ingredients have a bit of flour mix through them, pour the egg on top and almost fully combine the dough. Place the bowl into its secure position in the mixer and, using a dough hook attachment, knead the dough on a medium speed for 10 minutes.

Lightly grease a large bowl and transfer the dough to it, cover loosely with greased cling film (plastic wrap) and leave to prove in a warm spot for about 1 hour until doubled in size.

Cut 8 x 10cm / 4in squares of parchment paper and place them, spread out, on a large baking sheet. Divide the dough into 8 balls, then place each one on a paper square. Cover with the same cling film and return to the warm spot for a second prove, for about 1 hour until doubled in size. **>>>**

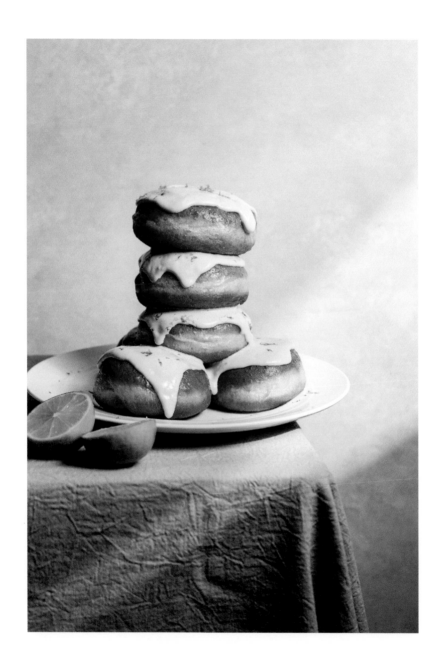

>>> Meanwhile, make the glaze by whipping the coconut milk, cream cheese and coconut sugar using a stand mixer or electric hand-whisk. Taste, add a little lime juice if you feel it needs it, then transfer to a bowl, cover and place in the fridge until needed.

Add the oil to a large, heavy-based saucepan (or deep fryer) and heat to 160°C / 320°F (check with a cooking thermometer). As soon as the oil is ready, carefully lower a few doughnuts in, by lifting them on their square (which will go into the oil too – this avoids you damaging the shape), and fry for 3–4 minutes on each side, gently flipping over with a slotted metal spoon. Transfer to a cooling rack, with a baking tray (pan) underneath to catch the oil. The paper squares will naturally separate from the dough as it fries, so just lift them out once loose. Repeat with the remaining doughnuts and leave to cool completely.

Pour the glaze over the cooled doughnuts and sprinkle the toasted desiccated (shredded) coconut on top, if you like, along with some lime zest. Doughnuts go stale pretty quickly, so it's best to eat them all up immediately.

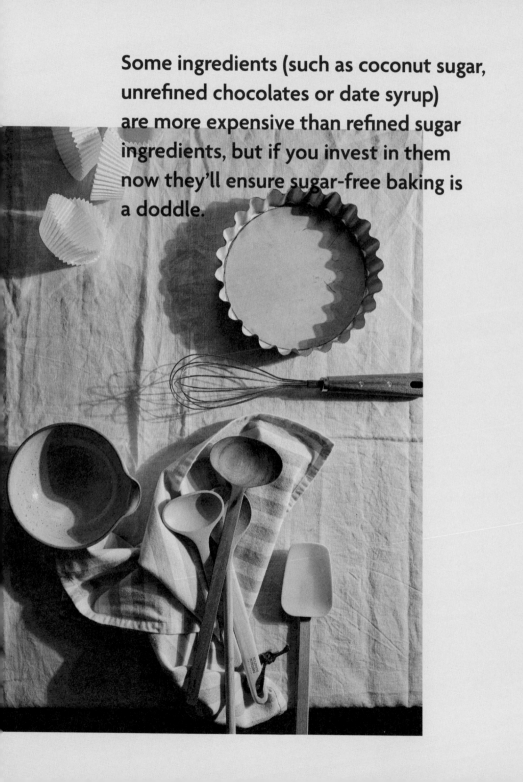

Some ingredients (such as coconut sugar, unrefined chocolates or date syrup) are more expensive than refined sugar ingredients, but if you invest in them now they'll ensure sugar-free baking is a doddle.

Miso & Sesame Peaches

\\\

SERVES 4

4 peaches
2 tbsp white miso
juice of 1 lemon
1 tsp coconut sugar, sifted
drizzle of sesame oil
1 tbsp toasted sesame seeds
 and some fresh mint,
 to serve (optional)

Preheat the oven to 200°C / 400°F / gas mark 6.

Halve the peaches and remove the stones, then place on a baking tray (pan).

Mix the miso and lemon juice in a small bowl, then spread this over the peach halves. Sprinkle over the coconut sugar, then bake on the top shelf of the oven for 30 minutes until tender and caramelized.

Drizzle over some sesame oil and return to the oven for a final 10 minutes.

Sprinkle over the sesame seeds and tear some fresh mint on top, to serve, if you like.

/ These are quite 'savoury', so either serve with yoghurt or the Mango Frozen Yoghurt, opposite, or serve as part of a summer feast (they are great cooked on a BBQ or grill too) instead of chutney.

Mango Frozen Yoghurt

**MAKES ABOUT 800ML /
3½ CUPS**

650g / 1lb 7oz mango flesh
1 x 410g / 14oz can
  (1⅔ cups) evaporated
  (not condensed) milk
140g / ¾ cup Greek strained
  yoghurt
2 tbsp runny honey
pinch of sea salt

Add all the ingredients to a food processor and blitz until very smooth. You'll have to do this in batches, so just make sure each batch has a bit of liquid in it to help blitz easily.

Once you have a large bowl of smooth liquid, pass it through a fine sieve into a freezer-safe, sealable container.

Freeze for 2 hours, then remove and blitz up again, this time in a jug blender for ease, to help smoothen the frozen yoghurt during the freezing process.

Return to the freezer for another 2 hours, blitz again, then repeat a third time.

Store in the freezer for up to 1 month. To serve, either bring it out to sit at room temperature for 10 minutes then blitz to soften, or let it sit at room temperature for about 30 minutes and scoop straight from the container.

/ **You can also churn the mixture in an ice-cream machine instead of as outlined above.**

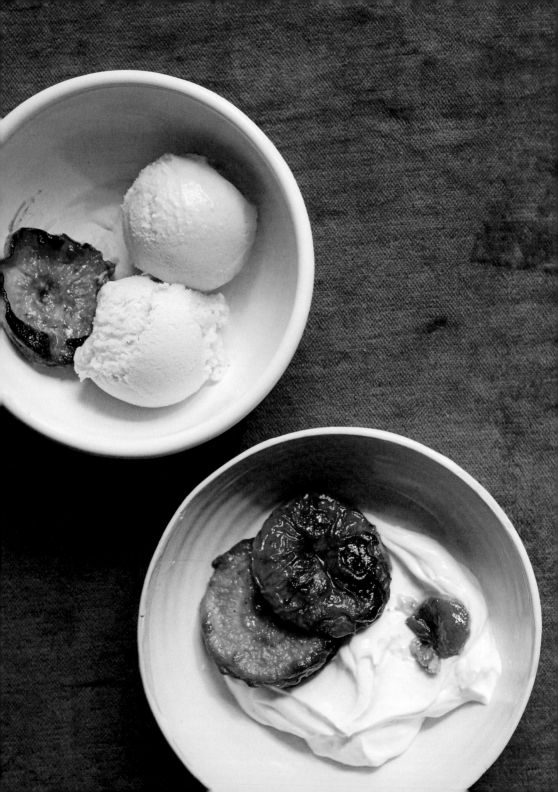

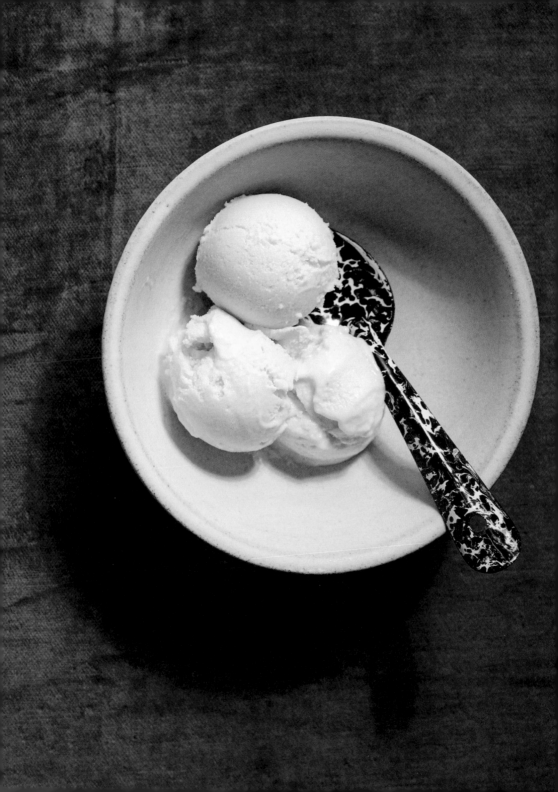

Cacao & Cherry Cheesecake

SERVES 8–10

BASE

160g / 4½ tbsp butter, plus
  extra for greasing
2 tbsp runny honey
300g / 10½oz plain oat cakes
½ tsp sea salt

FILLING

5 tbsp raw cacao powder
5 tbsp boiling water
100g / 3½oz xylitol
600g / 2⅔ cups cream cheese
300ml / 1¼ cups double
  (heavy) cream
150g / 1 cup frozen cherries,
  defrosted

TOPPING

raw cacao powder, for dusting
fresh cherries (keep stalks on)

Very lightly grease a 20cm / 8in loose-bottomed round cake tin (pan) and line with parchment paper.

Melt the butter and honey for the base in a small saucepan, then remove from the heat and set aside. Add the oatcakes and salt to a food processor and pulse until broken down into crumbs. Add the butter and honey mixture to the processor and pulse again until combined. Transfer the mixture to the base of the lined cake tin, levelling it out and pressing down with the back of a spoon to compress. Transfer to the freezer while you prepare the filling.

To make the filling, add the cacao powder and boiling water to a large mixing bowl and mix to a paste. Add the xylitol and cream cheese then, using an electric hand-whisk, mix to combine well until fluffy. Add the cream and continue to whip until further combined and reaching soft peaks. Fold through the defrosted cherries (and their juice), then spread out evenly on top of the set biscuit base, levelling out as you go. Cover, then place the cheesecake in the fridge and leave to set overnight.

Carefully remove the cheesecake from the cake tin, dust over a little cacao powder through a fine sieve, then add the whole cherries to the top to serve.

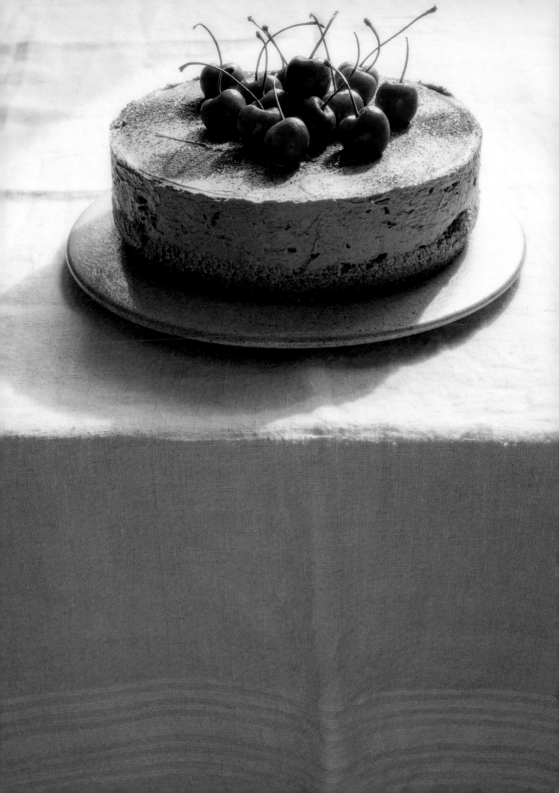

Mint Chocolate Mousse

SERVES 2

80g / 3oz 100% raw
   cacao chocolate (I use
   Montezuma's Absolute
   Black), broken into pieces
½ tsp mint extract
2 tbsp full-fat milk
4 eggs, separated
15g / ½oz xylitol
raw cacao powder, for dusting
fresh mint, to serve (optional)

Melt the chocolate, either in the microwave in 15-second bursts, or in a heatproof bowl set over a pan of simmering water, making sure the base of the bowl is not touching the water. Set aside to cool for about 20 minutes, stirring occasionally to keep it loose.

Add the mint extract and milk to the egg yolks in a bowl. Mix well to combine, then set aside.

Whip up the egg whites with an electric hand-whisk to soft peaks, then add the xylitol and whisk again briefly until you have glossy, stiff peaks.

Once the chocolate has cooled to lukewarm, add the yolky mixture to it and vigorously stir to combine. The mixture will loosen up.

Add one-third of the whisked egg whites to the chocolate bowl and whisk very quickly and vigorously to combine the two.

Next, add half the chocolate mixture to the egg whites and gently fold with a spatula to avoid losing the air in the whites. Once combined, add the remaining chocolate mixture and repeat the gentle folding action to incorporate all the ingredients. Transfer to 2 serving glasses and sprinkle with cacao powder.

Transfer to the fridge and let set for 5 hours, or overnight. Serve with some fresh mint on top, if you like.

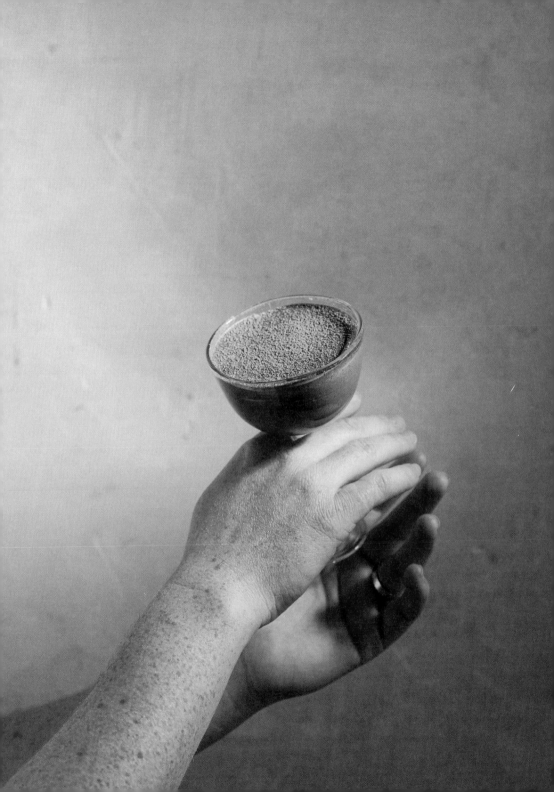

Coffee, Date & Pecan Cake

SERVES 8–10

2 tbsp hot milk

3 tbsp instant coffee granules

200g / 1½ cups self-raising (self-rising) flour

2 tsp bicarbonate of soda (baking soda)

180ml / ¾ cup groundnut oil

3 eggs

140g / 7 tbsp date syrup

80g / 3oz pecan halves, half roughly chopped and half saved for the top

140g / 5oz dates, pitted and roughly chopped

COFFEE CREAM

2 tbsp instant coffee granules

2 tbsp hot milk

200ml / ¾ cup double (heavy) cream

Preheat the oven to 170°C / 330°F / gas mark 3½. Line a non-stick 900g / 2lb loaf tin (pan) with parchment paper.

Add the hot milk and coffee granules to a small bowl and mix to dissolve and combine. In a large mixing bowl, put the flour, bicarbonate of soda (baking soda), oil, eggs, date syrup and the dissolved coffee mixture and, using an electric hand-whisk, whisk just briefly to combine; you don't want to overmix.

Once combined, fold through the chopped pecans and the dates, then pour into the prepared loaf tin. Smooth the top slightly and decorate the top with the pecan halves, in any way you like.

Bake on the middle shelf of the oven for 1 hour, or until risen, browned and cooked through (a skewer or knife inserted into the middle will come out clean). Place the cake in its tin on a cooling rack for 20 minutes, then turn the cake out and let cool completely.

While the cake is cooling, mix the coffee granules and hot milk to dissolve, then add the cream and whip to almost stiff peaks. Serve the cake with dollops of coffee cream on the side.

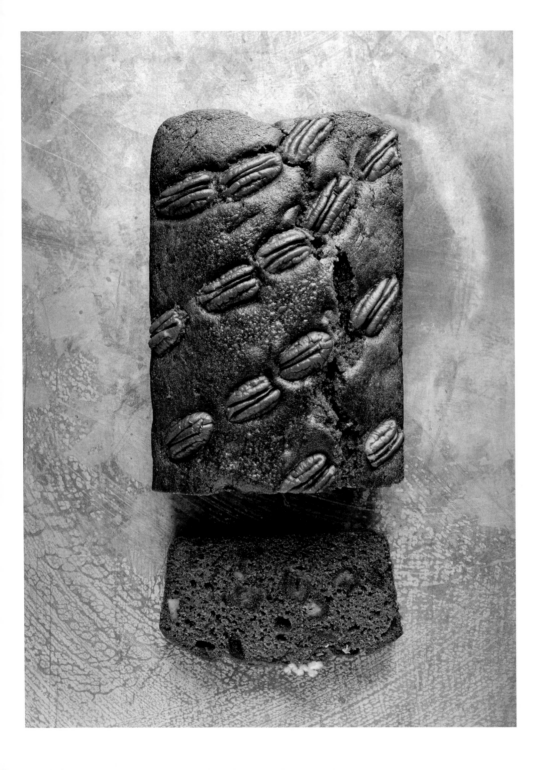

Carrot Cake

SERVES 8–10

butter, for greasing

190g / 1½ cups minus 1 tbsp
self-raising (self-rising)
flour

160g / ¾ cup plus 1 tbsp
coconut sugar, sifted

½ tsp sea salt

1 tsp ground cinnamon

1 tsp ground mixed spice

½ tsp ground nutmeg

1¼ tsp bicarbonate of soda
(baking soda)

190ml / ¾ cup plus 1 tbsp
vegetable oil

4 medium eggs

160g / 5¾oz carrots, coarsely
grated

40g / 4 tbsp chopped
hazelnuts

TOPPING

100g / scant ½ cup cream
cheese

100g / 6 tbsp strained Greek
yoghurt

zest of 1 lemon

1 tbsp maple syrup

2–3 tbsp chopped hazelnuts

Preheat the oven to 180°C / 350°F / gas mark 4. Grease a
20cm / 8in loose-bottomed round cake tin (pan) and line
with parchment paper.

Add all the cake ingredients, apart from the carrots
and hazelnuts, to a large mixing bowl and mix well to
combine, then fold through the carrots and hazelnuts.

Transfer the mixture to the prepared tin and bake on the
middle shelf of the oven for 50 minutes until cooked
through (a knife or skewer inserted into the middle will
come out clean).

Place the cake in its tin on a cooling rack for 15 minutes,
then turn the cake out and let cool completely.

For the topping, whip the cream cheese, yoghurt and
lemon zest together until smooth, then pile on top of the
fully cooled cake. Drizzle the maple syrup over the cream
cheese icing, then sprinkle over the chopped hazelnuts.

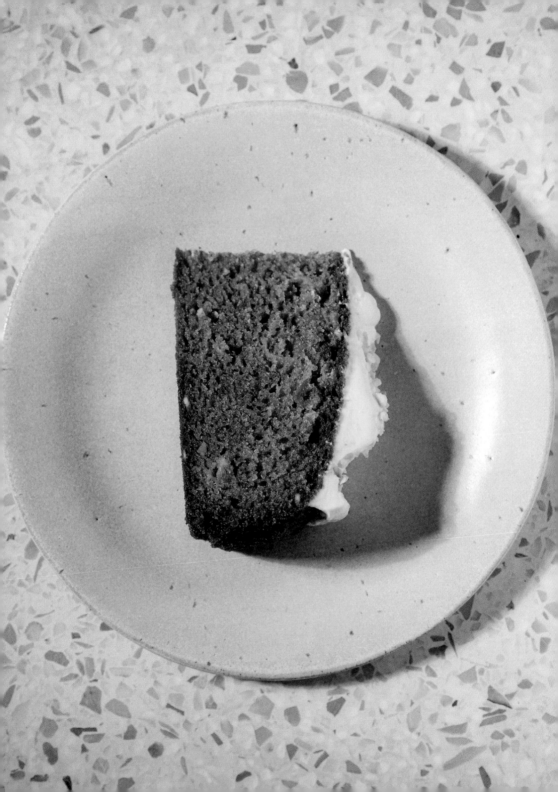

Baked Apples

SERVES 4

4 cooking / baking apples
20g / 1 tbsp raisins
20g / 1 tbsp walnuts, roughly
   chopped
pinch of ground nutmeg
4 large shards of cinnamon
   stick
20g / 1½ tbsp salted butter
single (light) cream, to serve

Preheat the oven to 200°C / 400°F / gas mark 6.

Core the apples and place in a baking dish.

Put the raisins, walnuts and nutmeg in a bowl and mix well to combine, then spoon into the cavities of each apple. Stick a piece of cinnamon into each cavity and squish a knob of butter into the filled cavities.

Bake for 30 minutes, then cover the dish with foil and bake for a further 20 minutes, or until the apples are very soft.

Let sit for a couple of minutes, then serve with cream.

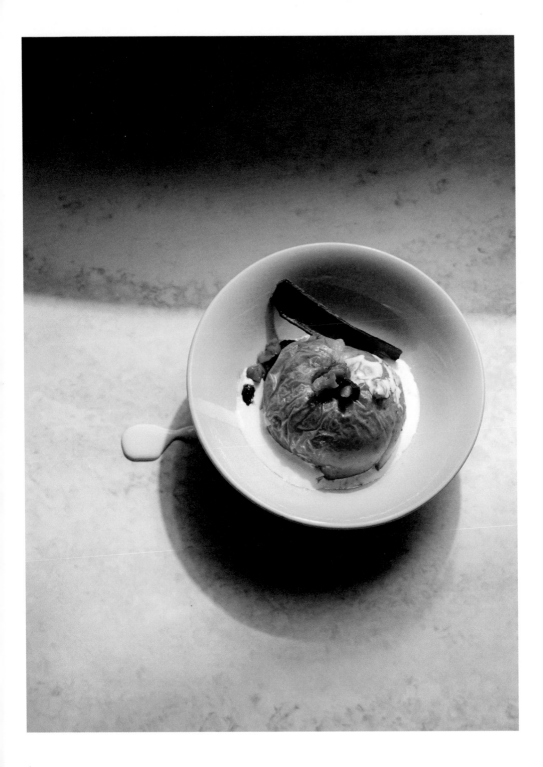

Bread & Butter Pudding

SERVES 6–8

60g / 4 tbsp butter, softened

6 slices of white bread

40g / ⅓ cup sultanas (golden
  raisins)

120g / scant ½ cup natural
  sugar jam (jelly) (I use St.
  Dalfour) or Fruit Compote
  (page 27)

350ml / 1½ cups full-fat milk

100ml / 7 tbsp double
  (heavy) cream, plus extra
  if needed

2 eggs

30g / 1oz xylitol

Grease a 1-litre / 4-cup oven dish with 10g / ¾ tbsp of the
butter, and use the rest to spread on one side of each bread
slice. Cut each slice in half diagonally, into 2 triangles.

Add a layer of bread to the base of the oven dish. Follow
with a sprinkling of sultanas (golden raisins) and a few
dots of jam (jelly) or Compote. Place a second layer of
bread on top, then follow with more sultanas and jam or
compote dots. Finish with the third layer of ingredients
and you should have reached the top of the baking dish.

Put the milk, cream, eggs and xylitol in a measuring jug
and whisk well with a fork to combine. Slowly pour over
the layered pudding, cover the whole dish and place in the
fridge to soak for 2 hours, or overnight.

Preheat the oven to 190°C / 375°F / gas mark 5. If the
liquid looks like it has all been absorbed, top up with
a little more cream, then transfer to the middle shelf
of the oven and bake for 40 minutes until golden on top
and set, but with a nice little wobble in the middle still.
Serve immediately.

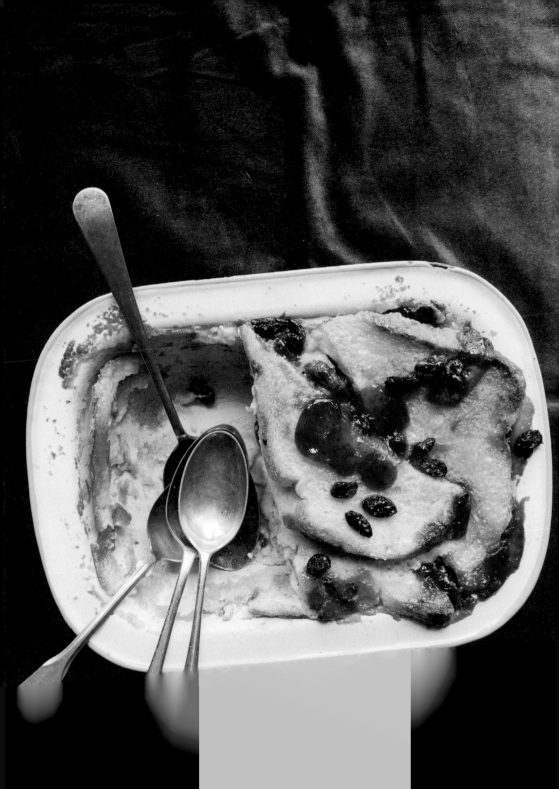

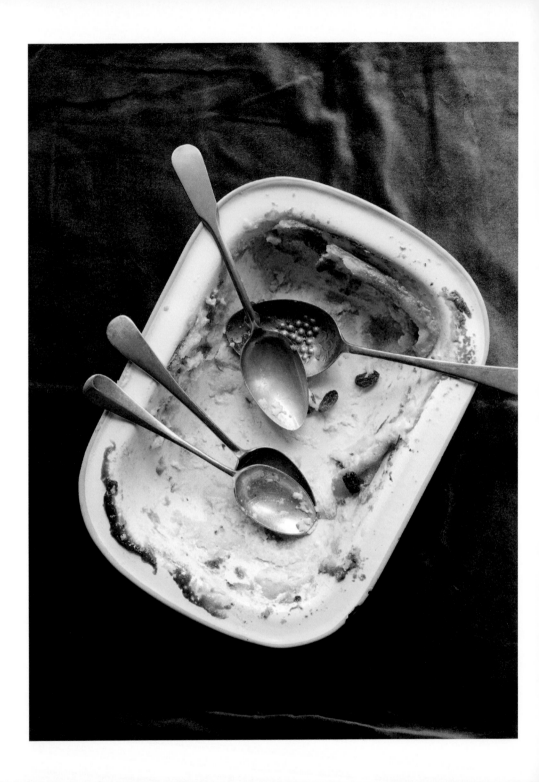

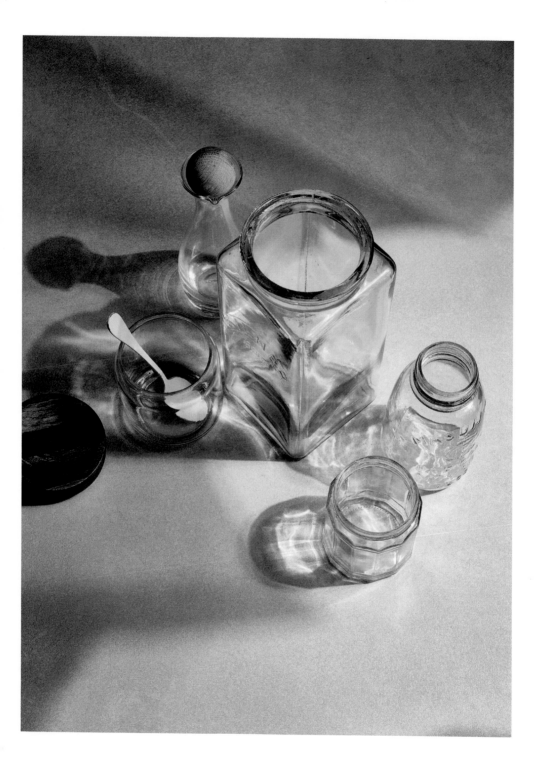

Apple & Date Cobblers

SERVES 4–6

10g / ¾ tbsp butter, softened,
   for greasing
1 Braeburn apple
1 Bramley apple
3 Medjool dates, pitted and
   finely chopped
pinch of ground nutmeg
double (heavy) cream, clotted
   cream or yoghurt, to serve

TOPPING
100g / ¾ cup plain
   (all-purpose) flour
¼ tsp sea salt
40g / scant ¼ cup coconut
   sugar, sifted
pinch of ground cinnamon
70g / scant ⅓ cup butter,
   softened
20g / scant ¼ cup porridge
   oats

Preheat the oven to 200°C / 400°F / gas mark 6.

Using your fingers, lightly grease the base and sides of
4 x 200ml / ¾ cup ovenproof dishes or ramekins with the
softened butter.

Core the apples, then chop into small pieces and add to a
large mixing bowl. Add the dates, along with a good pinch
of nutmeg. Toss to combine well and divide between the
prepared oven dishes.

For the topping, add the flour, salt, sugar, cinnamon
and butter to a food processor and briefly pulse until
the mixture goes slightly past the crumb stage and into
chunky lumps. Fold through the oats, then divide between
the dishes on top of the fruit. (The cobbler topping is
meant to be lumpier than a crumble topping.)

Bake for 50 minutes until golden and bubbling a little
around the edges.

Remove from the oven and let sit for 5 minutes, then serve
with cream or yoghurt.

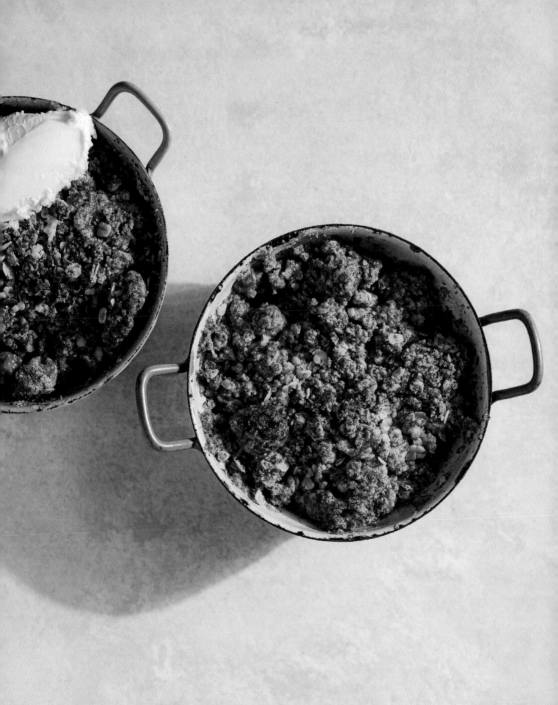

Mini Profiteroles

MAKES ABOUT
20 PROFITEROLES
40g / 3 tbsp unsalted butter
1 tbsp xylitol
¼ tsp sea salt
130ml / 8 tbsp plus 2 tsp
    water
80g / ⅔ cup minus 1 tbsp
    plain (all-purpose) flour
2 eggs, beaten

FILLING & TOPPING
200g / scant 1 cup double
    (heavy) cream
70g / 2½oz 100% raw
    cacao chocolate (I use
    Montezuma's Absolute
    Black), broken into pieces

Place the butter, xylitol, salt and water in a medium saucepan on a low heat to melt the butter, then bring to a simmer. As soon as it is simmering, reduce the heat and add the flour. Stir constantly for about 2 minutes with a wooden spoon until the mixture starts to come away from the sides of the pan, then remove from the heat.

Transfer the mixture to a large mixing bowl and add a very small slosh of the beaten egg, whisking it in immediately with an electric hand-whisk. Whisk in the remaining egg gradually until you have a smooth and shiny dough. Cover the dough (directly on top of the dough rather than the bowl) with cling film (plastic wrap), then transfer to the fridge to rest for 30 minutes.

Preheat the oven to 220°C / 425°F / gas mark 7.

Spoon the dough into a piping bag and pipe cherry-tomato-sized balls onto a lined baking tray (pan). Bake on the top shelf of the oven for 12–15 minutes until risen, golden and puffed. Remove from the oven and use a skewer to poke a small hole in the side of each profiterole so the steam can escape and help them cool, keeping their shape. Leave to cool completely. >>>

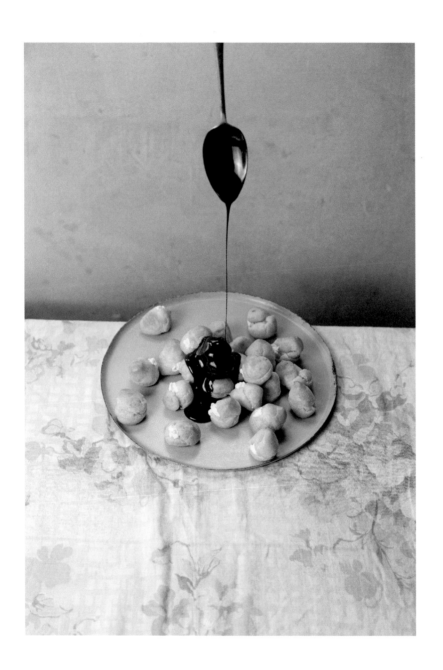

>>> For the filling, whip the cream to stiff peaks, then add to another piping bag, make a slightly larger hole in the side of each profiterole, insert the piping bag and gently fill with cream.

For the topping, melt the chocolate (either in a microwave, for about three 15-second bursts, or in a small heatproof bowl set over a pan of simmering water, making the sure the base of the bowl doesn't touch the water), then drizzle the melted chocolate over the profiteroles.

Let the chocolate cool slightly, then serve.

Lemon Crêpe Cake

\\

SERVES 8–10

CRÊPES (MAKES 12–15)

300g / 2¼ cups plain
  (all-purpose) flour

4 eggs

500ml / 2 cups full-fat milk

1 tsp vanilla extract

2 tsp lemon extract

½ tsp sea salt

butter, for frying

LEMON FILLING

780g / 3½ cups cream cheese

500g / 2¼ cups mascarpone

zest and juice of 6 lemons

3 tbsp xylitol

Whisk all the crêpe ingredients, except the butter, together in a large bowl until very smooth, then cover and transfer to the fridge to rest for 1 hour, or overnight.

Prepare the crêpe-making station, as you're going to make about 15 in one go. Place a 25cm / 10in non-stick frying pan on the hob, with a dinner plate on the side and a knob of butter in a bowl, also on the side. You'll need about a 70ml / 4–5 tbsp vessel or ladle for scooping the right amount of batter.

Heat the frying pan on a low–medium heat. Add a small knob of butter (you don't want the pan too oiled) and, once melted, add the first dollop of batter, rolling the pan in a circular motion to make a crêpe. Fry gently for about 2 minutes, then flip and cook on the other side for 30–60 seconds. Transfer to the plate and repeat with the remaining batter, adding a little butter occasionally. (If the butter burns, wipe it out with a clean cloth or kitchen paper. The temperature of the pan will increase the longer it is on the hob, so be aware and manage the heat.)

Leave the cooked crêpes to cool completely while you make the lemon filling. Whisk all the ingredients together, reserving the zest of one of the lemons to decorate the top. (Store the filling in the fridge if you're not assembling the cake imminently.) **>>>**

>>> Place one crêpe on a cake stand or serving plate.
Pile on a scoop of the lemon filling, spread out almost
to the edge, and place another crêpe on top. Repeat this
layering process until you reach the final crêpe, and pile
an extra serving of lemon filling on top. Transfer to the
fridge to set for about 2 hours.

Just before serving, top with the reserved lemon zest.
Cut into slices, as you would a cake, to serve.

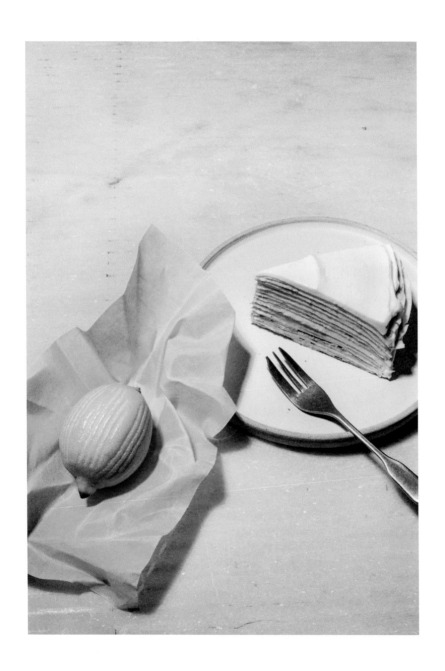

Melon, Lime & Honey Granita

SERVES 4–6

150ml / 10 tbsp water
2 tbsp honey
zest and juice of 2 limes
1 cantaloupe melon, skin
  and seeds discarded
  (400g / 14oz flesh)

Add all the ingredients to a food processor and blitz until smooth.

Transfer the mixture to a freezer container and place, uncovered, in the freezer for 3 hours, breaking up the granita every 30 minutes, by scraping the mixture with a fork.

Store in the freezer, covered, for up to 1 month, and just give it a fresh scrape when you're ready to serve.

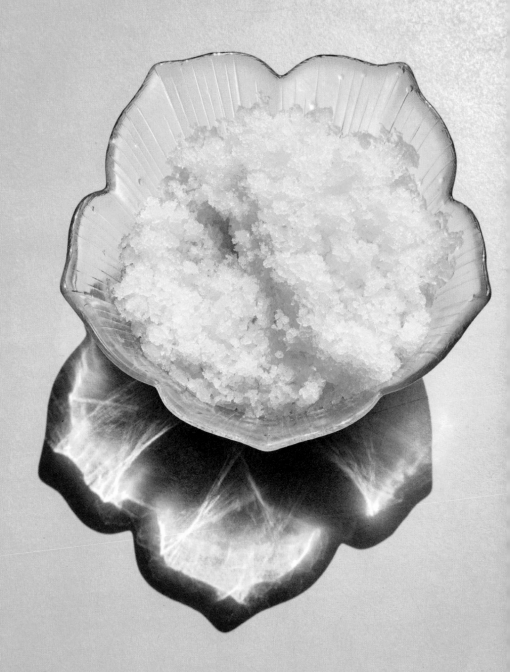

Layered Fruit Pots

\\\\\\\\\\\\\\\\\\\\\\\\\\\\\\\\\\\\

SERVES 4

200g / scant 1 cup double
(heavy) cream
120g / ½ cup plain yoghurt
zest of 1 lemon
100g / 3½oz Fruit Compote
(page 27)
40g / 4 tbsp chopped
hazelnuts
2 bananas, sliced
seasonal fruit, to serve

Whip the cream into a large mixing bowl until it reaches stiff peaks, then fold through the yoghurt and lemon zest.

Divide almost all of the Fruit Compote between the bases of 4 x 200ml / ¾ cup glasses, then top with a generous spoonful of the cream mixture (use half of it), half the nuts, all of the banana slices, then top with the rest of the cream mixture. Finish with a dollop of the remaining Fruit Compote and hazelnuts. (You can also add some freshly sliced, seasonal fruit throughout the glass too, if you wish.)

Serve immediately, or cover and refrigerate until needed, removing the pots from the fridge 15 minutes before serving.

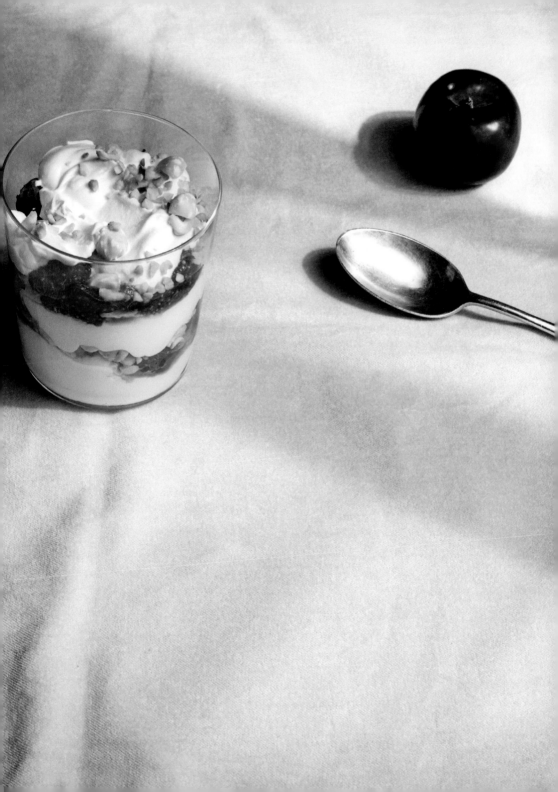

Banana & Date Smoothie

SERVES 1
1 banana
2 tbsp almond butter
3 dates
1 tsp raw cacao powder
150ml / ⅔ cup oat milk
handful of ice

Add all the ingredients to a NutriBullet or high-powered blender and blitz until smooth. Serve immediately.

Pink Power Smoothie

SERVES 1

90g / ⅔ cup frozen mixed
  berries
1 tbsp beetroot powder
handful of fresh spinach
150ml / 10 tbsp milk of your
  choice
50ml / 3½ tbsp water
juice of ½ lemon
handful of ice

Add all the ingredients to a NutriBullet or high-powered
blender and blitz until smooth. Serve immediately.

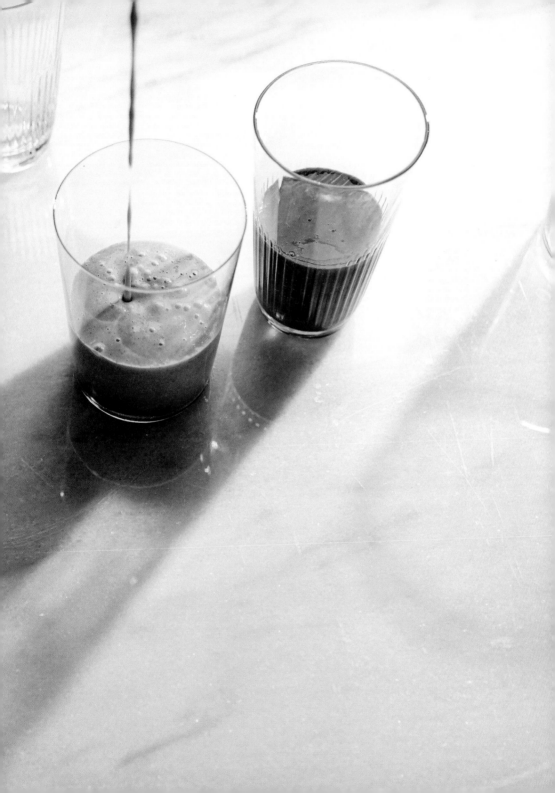

Malt Milk Pops

MAKES 8 ICE LOLLIES

1 x 410g / 14oz can
  (1⅔ cups) evaporated
  (not condensed) milk
200g / 1 cup Greek strained
  yoghurt
50g / 2½ tbsp malt extract
30g / 1½ tbsp date syrup
1 tsp vanilla extract
2 tbsp runny honey
pinch of sea salt

Add all the ingredients to a NutriBullet or high-powered blender and blitz to combine.

Pour the mixture into ice-lolly moulds, then top with the lid and lolly sticks.

Freeze for 8 hours, or overnight, and store in the freezer for up to 1 month

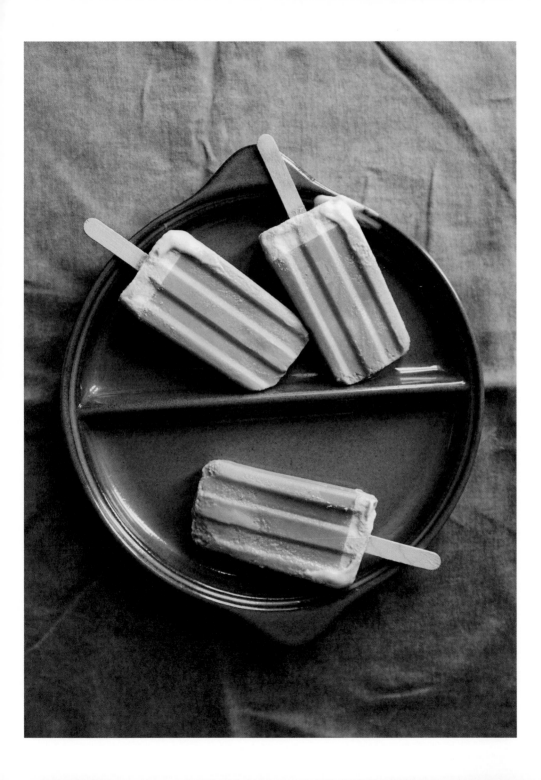

Mint, Ricotta & Nectarine Tartlets

MAKES 12 TARTLETS

2 nectarines, stoned and chopped, skin on (about 200g / 7oz flesh)
juice of 1 orange
10g / ⅓oz mint leaves
80g / ⅓ cup ricotta
2 sheets of filo pastry
20g / 1½ tbsp butter, melted

Preheat the oven to 200°C / 400°F / gas mark 6.

Add the nectarines to a saucepan with the orange juice. Bring to the boil, then simmer for 10 minutes until the fruit is breaking down and the mixture is jammy. Remove from the heat and set aside.

Stack half the mint leaves (reserve the smallest leaves for decorating) and roll them up together, then very finely slice. Mix through the ricotta in a small bowl.

Cut out 36 x 7cm / 2¾in (approximately) squares of filo pastry, placing them in a slightly damp kitchen towel as you work, to prevent them from drying out.

Brush each cavity of a 12-hole mini muffin or tartlet baking tray (pan) with melted butter.

Each tartlet will be made up of 3 layered squares, all brushed with butter. Lay one square on the work surface and brush lightly with butter, then add another square on top, slightly rotating the angle so the points of the square are all exposed around the edge. Brush that too, and top with a final square, also slightly angled and brushed. Pick up the three-layered tartlet case and push it gently into one of the baking tray cavities. Repeat with the remaining filo squares to make 12 tartlet cases. Divide the minty ricotta mixture between the cases, then top with the nectarine.

Bake on the middle shelf of the oven for 20 minutes, until the pastry is crisp and golden. Transfer the tray to a cooling rack and leave to cool fully before removing the tartlets and serving, topped with the reserved mint leaves.

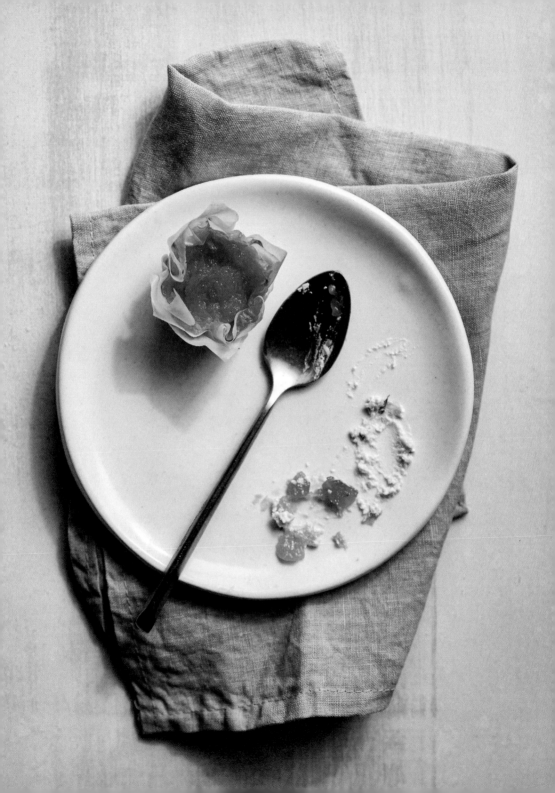

Stone Fruit Slices

\\

MAKES 9 SLICES

ROUGH PUFF PASTRY

110g / ¾ cup plus 1½ tbsp
  self-raising (self-rising)
  flour, plus extra for dusting
70g / ⅓ cup minus 1 tsp
  unsalted butter, chilled
  and diced
70ml / 4½ tbsp cold water
1 egg, beaten

FILLING

2 plums, nectarines, peaches
  or apricots (whatever is
  in season and ripe)
¼ tsp ground cinnamon
¼ tsp sea salt
zest of 1 lemon
2 tsp coconut sugar, sifted

To make the rough puff pastry, add the flour, butter and water to a mixing bowl and start to bring it together with your hands. Once the mixture has pretty much come together (big lumps of butter are fine), tip it out onto a lightly floured work surface, toss a bit more flour on top (and on the rolling pin) and start rolling out, dusting any exposed clumps of butter with more flour as you go.

Roll the dough out to a rectangle about 1cm / ⅜in thick, then fold up the bottom third over the central third of the rectangle, then fold the top third over the centre, so you have 3 equal layers.

Roll out again (keep using a bit of flour if any butter is exposed) to another 1cm / ⅜in thick rectangle, then repeat the folding. Do the rolling and folding process a third time. Put the folded pastry in a freezer bag and place in the fridge to chill for 1 hour, or until needed.

Halve, stone and thinly slice the fruit for the filling, then add to a bowl and toss with the cinnamon, salt, lemon zest and half the coconut sugar. Leave to macerate while the pastry is resting. >>>

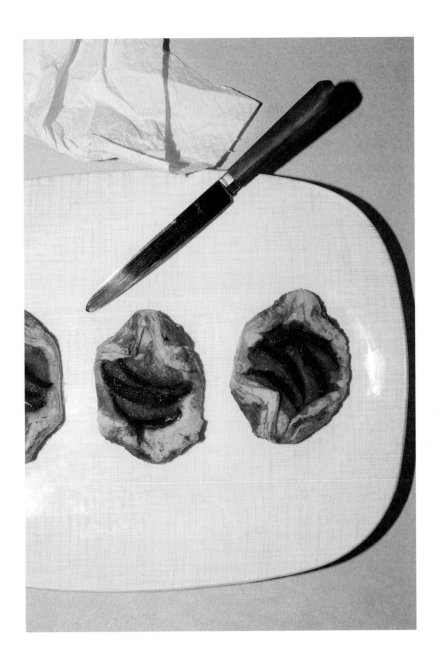

>>> Preheat the oven to 200°C / 400°F / gas mark 6.

Roll out the pastry into a rectangle about 27 x 20cm / 10½ x 8in, and 5mm–1cm / ⅛–⅜in thick, and cut into 9 rectangles. Place 3 or 4 slices of fruit in the centre of each, then fold in the corners over the fruit until they almost meet. Brush the pastry edges with the beaten egg, then sprinkle over the remaining sugar.

Place on a lined baking tray (pan) and bake for 25 minutes until golden, bubbling and puffed up. Leave to cool for 5 minutes before serving just as they are, or as a dessert with yoghurt.

Xylitol tastes and looks exactly like common white sugar, but contains fewer calories and doesn't create spikes in blood-sugar levels.

Xylitol can be processed from trees like birch or from a plant fibre called xylan. If you can't get hold of xylitol, stevia is a similar natural sweetner that you can use as a substitute.

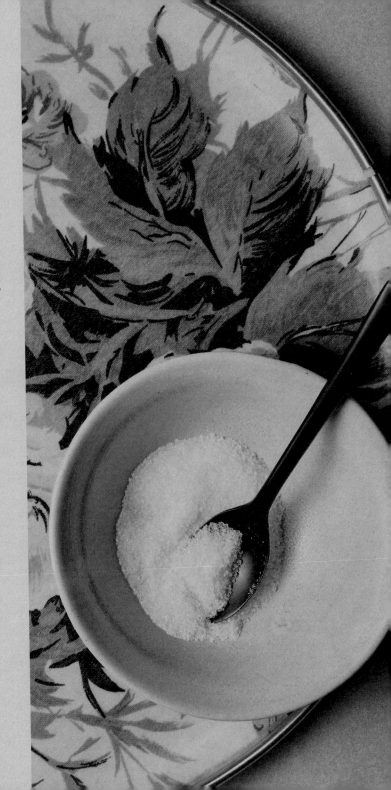

Raisin, Cranberry & Orange Florentines

\\\\\\\\\\\\\\\\\\\\\\\\\\\\\\\\\\\\

MAKES 8–10 FLORENTINES

50g / scant ½ cup dried
  cranberries
30g / 3 tbsp sultanas
  (golden raisins)
100g / 1¼ cups flaked
  (slivered) almonds
zest of 1 orange
¼ tsp sea salt
1 tbsp plain (all-purpose)
  flour
30g / 2 tbsp butter, melted
1 tsp orange extract
1 tsp double (heavy) cream
1 tsp honey
1 tsp xylitol

Preheat the oven to 180°C / 360°F / gas mark 4. Line 2 large baking trays (pans) with parchment paper.

Add the cranberries, sultanas (golden raisins), almonds, half the orange zest, salt and flour to a large mixing bowl and stir well to combine and coat.

Put the melted butter, orange extract, cream, honey and xylitol into a small saucepan and let melt, but not bubble. Add the melted ingredients to the mixing bowl and stir to combine.

Using a dessertspoon, scoop up a portion of the mixture and place on a prepared baking tray, gently flattening it and making sure there are no holes; you want all the ingredients to be touching. Repeat with the remaining mixture, using both trays, keeping a good 5cm / 2in space between each Florentine.

Bake for 10–12 minutes, then remove and leave to cool for 20 minutes, still on the baking trays.

Serve immediately or store in an airtight container at room temperature for up to 3 days.

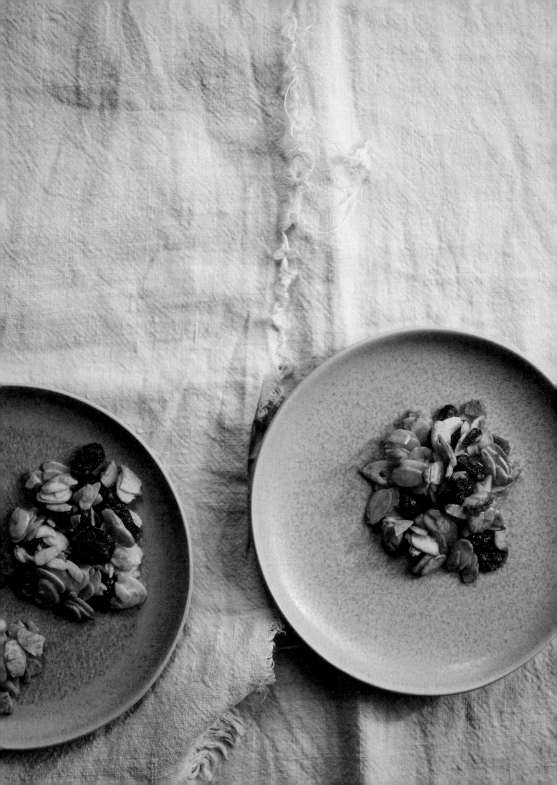

Fridge Bars

MAKES 8–10 BARS

150g / 1 cup mixed dried
   berries (cranberries,
   sultanas, raisins, cherries)
50g / ¼ cup chopped
   hazelnuts
60g / ½ cup roasted peanuts
70g / ½ cup pitted Medjool
   dates, chopped
30g / ⅓ cup porridge oats
30g / 1oz puffed brown rice
70g / 2½oz 100% raw
   cacao chocolate (I use
   Montezuma's Absolute
   Black), broken into pieces
60g / 4½ tbsp coconut oil
120g / ½ cup smooth peanut
   butter
100g / scant ½ cup almond
   butter

Line a 20cm / 8in square baking tin (pan) with
parchment paper.

Add the berries, hazelnuts, peanuts, dates, oats and
puffed rice to a large mixing bowl.

Put the chocolate, coconut oil, peanut butter and almond
butter in a small saucepan over a low heat and gently
melt until loose; don't worry if there are a few nut
butter lumps that won't break down. Pour over the dry
ingredients and fold together until fully combined, then
pile into the prepared tin, spreading the mixture out to
the edges and compressing with the back of a spoon.

Let cool to room temperature, then place in the fridge
for 3 hours to set.

Remove from the tin, cut into 8–10 bars and serve,
or store in an airtight container in the fridge.

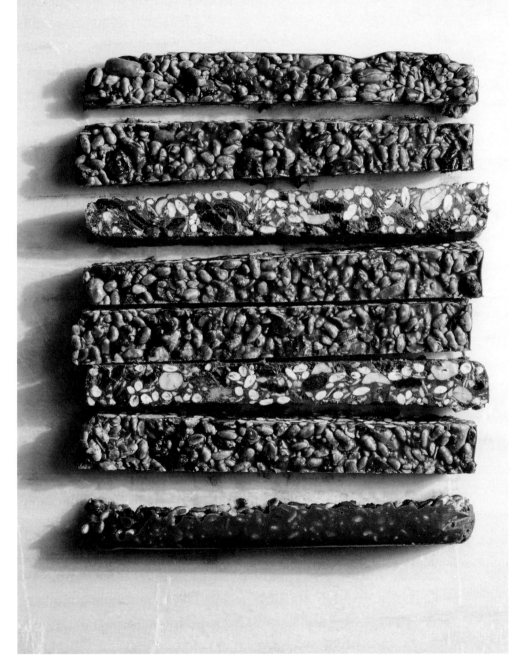

You can still treat yourself to chocolate while avoiding refined sugar – just be sure to buy 100% cacao.

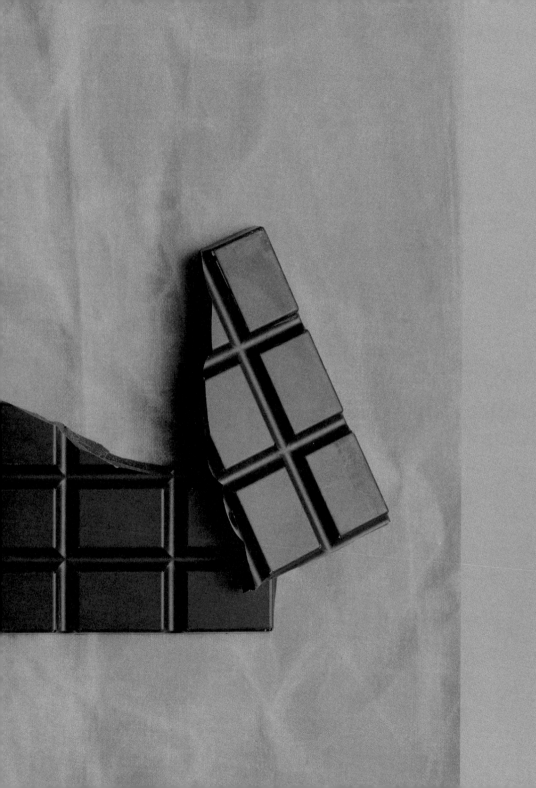

Almond, Lemon & Coconut Biscuits

MAKES 10 BISCUITS

50g / ¼ cup coconut sugar, sifted

110g / ½ cup salted butter, softened

1 tsp lemon extract

100g / ¾ cup plain (all-purpose) flour

100g / 1 cup ground almonds

30g / 5 tbsp desiccated (dried shredded) coconut

zest of 1 lemon

Line a large baking sheet with parchment paper.

Add the sugar, butter and lemon extract to a mixing bowl and mix thoroughly until fully combined and slightly paler. Add the flour and ground almonds and fold through until combined, being careful not to overwork the mixture.

Transfer the dough to a large, double layer of cling film (plastic wrap) laid out on a clean surface and briefly mould into a sausage shape.

Use the cling film to help mould and roll the dough into a sausage about 7cm / 2¾in diameter, and about 13cm / 5in long. Seal the cling film and tighten, making sure there are no air bubbles. Secure the ends and transfer to the freezer for 30 minutes to firm up. Mix the desiccated (shredded) coconut with the lemon zest and set aside.

Preheat the oven to 160°C / 325°F / gas mark 3.

Once the dough sausage is firm, slice into discs about 1cm / ⅜in thick and transfer to the prepared baking sheet. Sprinkle the coconut and lemon zest mixture on top of the biscuits, then bake on the top shelf of the oven for 25 minutes until golden on top.

Remove from the oven and leave to cool on the sheet for 15 minutes, before transferring to a cooling rack to cool completely.

Store in an airtight container for up to 5 days.

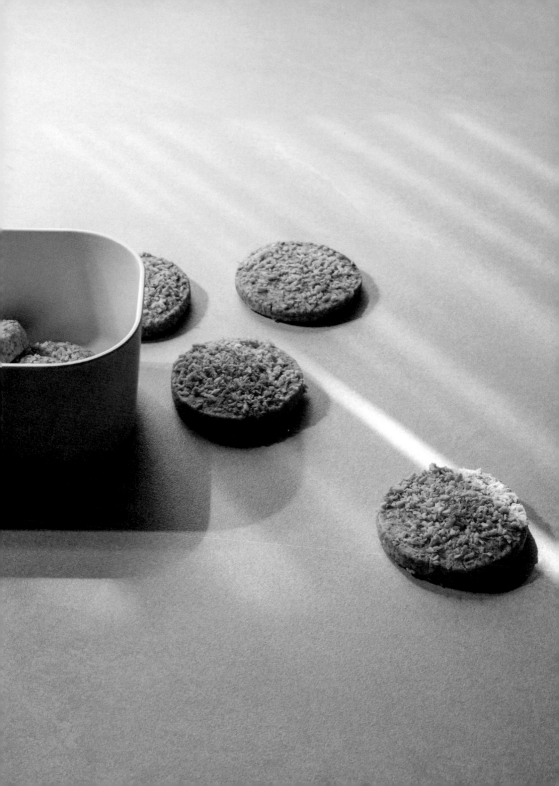

Rice Crispy Cakes

MAKES 12 CAKES

60g / 4½ tbsp unsalted butter

100g / 3½oz 100% raw
  cacao chocolate (I use
  Montezuma's Absolute
  Black), broken into pieces

¼ tsp sea salt

2 tbsp maple syrup

100g / 3½oz puffed brown
  rice

Add the butter, chocolate and salt to a small saucepan and gently melt, stirring often. Remove from the heat, then immediately stir in the maple syrup.

Put the puffed rice in a mixing bowl and pour over the melted mixture. Fold gently to coat all the cereal in the chocolate mixture.

Divide between 12 muffin cases and leave to cool completely.

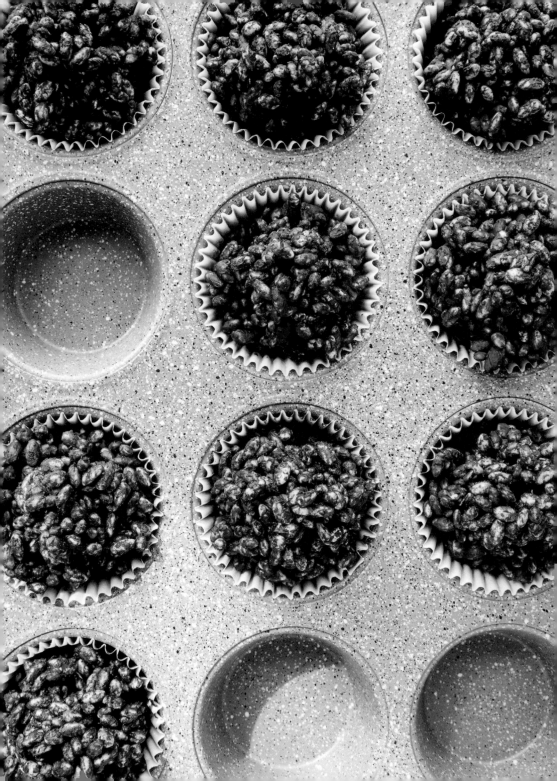

Snickers Bites

MAKES 10 BITES

10 Medjool dates
6 tbsp crunchy peanut butter
70g / 2½oz 100% raw
   cacao chocolate (I use
   Montezuma's Absolute
   Black), broken into pieces
flaky sea salt, to sprinkle

Using a small, sharp knife, make an incision down the length of each date. Remove and discard the stones, then fill each date with peanut butter. Place on a plate and transfer to the freezer for 10 minutes.

Before the end of the 10 minutes, place the chocolate in a microwave-safe mug or small bowl. Melt for 1 minute in 15-second bursts, stirring between each burst (or melt the chocolate in a heatproof bowl set over a pan of simmering water, making sure the bowl is not touching the water).

Dip each stuffed date, one at a time, in the melted chocolate (toothpicks and a teaspoon help here), place back on the plate and add a small sprinkling of sea salt on the top of each, before the chocolate solidifies.

Freeze for another 20 minutes, then devour or store in the freezer. They are best stored individually wrapped in a little parchment paper, in a lidded freezer container or bag.

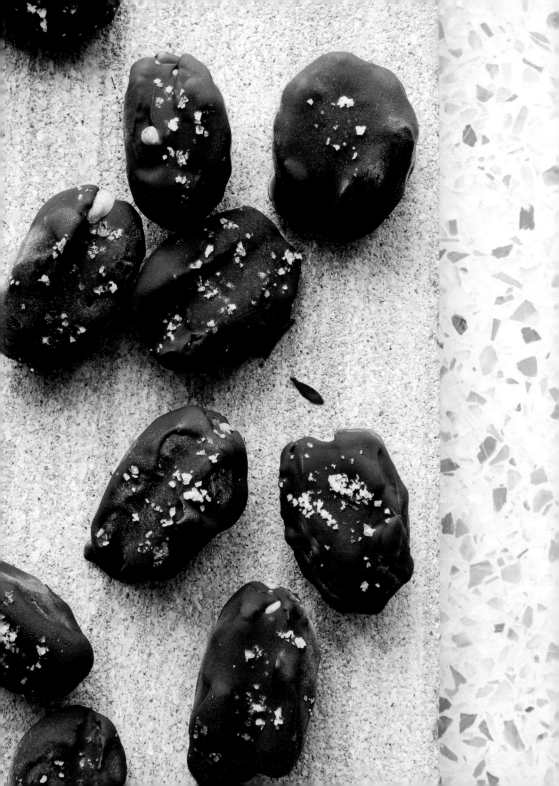

Fruit Jelly Sweets

6 gelatine sheets
200g / 7oz Fruit Compote
  (page 27)
200ml / ¾ cup apple juice
100ml / 7 tbsp water
1 tbsp runny honey

Add the gelatine sheets to a bowl of cold water and set aside to soften.

Meanwhile, add the Fruit Compote, apple juice and water to a NutriBullet or high-powered blender and blitz until very smooth. Transfer to a saucepan and bring almost to the boil, whisking often, then remove from the heat and let cool slightly for 5 minutes.

When the compote mixture is ready (you don't want to add gelatine to a boiling-hot mixture; it won't set), squeeze out the excess water from the gelatine sheets and whisk the gelatine through the fruit mixture to fully dissolve.

Pour the mixture onto a small, lipped non-stick baking tray (pan) and let cool. Once it is at room temperature, cover, transfer to the fridge and leave to set completely for at least 3 hours, or overnight.

Using a small, round pastry cutter or similar, cut the jelly into sweeties (or into squares to avoid wastage), then store in an airtight container in the fridge for up to 5 days.

/ You could split this recipe in half and make two different-flavoured jelly sweets with different-flavoured compotes.

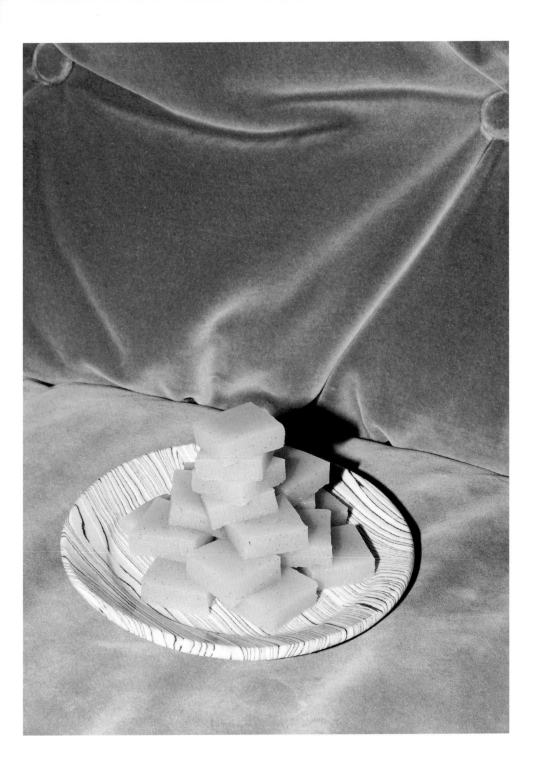

Some cheap supermarket honeys contain hidden refined sugars.

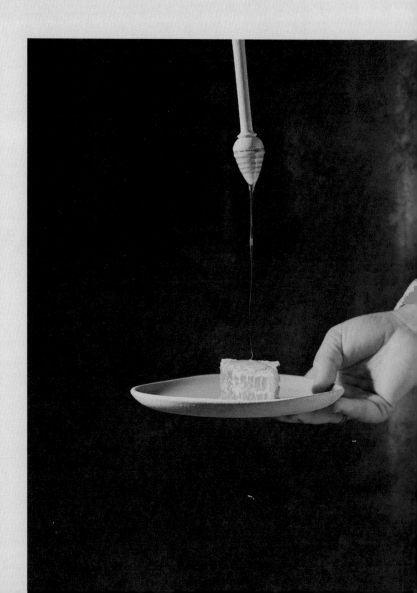